THE TOOL KIT FOR DENTAL RISK MANAGEMENT

Roy Lilley
and
Paul Lambden

Radcliffe Medical Press

Radcliffe Medical Press Ltd
18 Marcham Road
Abingdon
Oxon OX14 1AA
United Kingdom

www.radcliffe-oxford.com
The Radcliffe Medical Press electronic catalogue and online ordering facility.
Direct sales to anywhere in the world.

British Library Cataloguing in Publication Data

A catalogue record for this book is available from the British Library.

ISBN 1 85775 970 2

Typeset by Joshua Associates Ltd, Oxford
Printed and bound by TJ International Ltd, Padstow, Cornwall

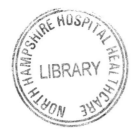

CONTENTS

PREFACE

NHS dentistry has undergone a quiet revolution. What started as a universal service, interwoven with the NHS, became de-coupled from its beginnings to the point where, in some parts of the country, it became difficult or impossible to find a dentist still willing to practise within the terms of the NHS.

In the mid-nineties dentistry and government fell out. For some there were points of principle to be settled. For others it was little more than an industrial dispute. The row focused, primarily, on dentists' remuneration. Government seemed determined to rein in NHS dental costs and practitioners were equally determined that a quality service should be preserved against a background of rising costs. It is probably true that there was some profiteering in the system, it is equally true that NHS inflation in raw materials and operating costs took its toll.

The outcome had the severest impact on NHS patients. Dentists turned their backs on the public sector in their droves and progressively moved into private practice. Underpinned by a growing private dental insurance plan market, dentists consolidated private practice and the full-time NHS dentist became a rarity. Extraordinarily, there was no public outcry on the scale that might have been predicted. Nevertheless, the impact on the nation's dental health is probably yet to emerge.

The years of Conservative administrations, that oversaw the demise of NHS dentistry, came to an end with a Labour Government determined to modernise the NHS. Huge injections of resources are now promised and planned. The combination of a Labour administration committed to public service expansion and a booming economy means all sectors of the NHS should benefit. There is a re-affirmation to NHS dentistry. The blue-print for the development of health services over the next ten years was published in the summer of 2000. The NHS Plan.

The Plan sets out an ambitious future for NHS dentistry. It says:

> The Government is firmly committed to making high quality NHS dentistry available to all who want it by September 2001. The initiatives we have taken since 1997 have already made a real difference but more needs to be done. In future, NHS Direct will help direct patients to NHS dentistry. The Government will fund more dental access centres and improvements to dental practices. It will reward dentists' commitment to the NHS and foster better quality services for patients, making NHS dentistry a modern and truly national service again. Health authorities will take the lead in delivering the changes which patients expect.

It seems dentistry is to come full circle . . .

Whilst all this medico-political turmoil has been going on, what has happened to dentistry? Advances in technology have, unarguably, improved treatments. Some well publicised disasters have focused the profession on the role and use of anaesthetics. Costs have risen and the public has become more demanding. Out of hours practice is now more common, so too is a patient's willingness to sue the dentist if he or she feels in some way aggrieved.

Is this a good time to be a dentist? Well, certainly the backdrop has changed and there are interesting options on the horizon. But, as the Chinese proverb says, 'Pray you never live in interesting times'!

This book intends to look at the practise of dentistry in the new environment. An environment where dental surgeries in supermarkets will be commonplace and health authorities will use some of their windfall, new funding, to provide dental services in health centres and general practitioner's premises. An environment where dentists can play a part in developing and improving the health of communities through the new Health Improvement Programmes. An environment where dentists have, undoubtedly, improved their practice, invested in their skills and moved their profession forward. An environment where some dentists have doggedly remained committed to the NHS and others now work solely in private practice.

Wherever dentistry is practised there are risks. Risks to patients, to dentists, to staff, to premises and to reputations. Risk management is the skill of seeking out the risks and managing them by simple common-sense measures, which provide peace of mind and safety.

As dentistry is, once again, set to be placed centre stage, risk management takes on a new significance. Risk management is not rocket science, neither is it something that can be left to someone else. Risk management is the professional response, by professional people working in a fast changing environment.

This book sets out to address the issues, help you find the answers and to prove that management can be fun . . .

Roy Lilley
Paul Lambden
August 2001

ABOUT THE AUTHORS

Roy Lilley is a former businessman, NHS Trust chair and vice-chair of a health authority, and has just completed a four year rotation as a visiting fellow at the Management School, Imperial College. He is the creator of the highly successful Tool Kit series.

Roy is a frequent commentator and broadcaster on health and social issues, a regular on TV and radio and he writes for national newspapers, magazines and periodicals on NHS and related issues. He speaks on platforms in the UK, mainland Europe and the US on social and health issues and the management of change.

His aim with the Tool Kit books is to take topical issues that challenge and change the NHS and to help prepare those most involved for their impact in a straightforward, common-sense way.

Dr Paul Lambden, BSc MB BS BDS FDSRCS MRCS LRCP DRCOG MHSM, graduated in dentistry, medicine and science at Guy's Hospital, London. After working initially in oral surgery and gaining his Fellowship of the Royal College of Surgeons, he entered general medical and dental practice, continuing the two for 15 years. He was also a clinical tutor at St Bartholomew's Hospital, London.

In 1992 he left practice to become the Chief Executive of a whole district NHS trust and also worked as a specialist adviser to the all-party Parliamentary Health Select Committee. He is now the Medical and Dental Principal of the St Paul International Insurance Company Ltd.

Paul is a regular writer on medical, health and management topics. He has appeared on many radio and television programmes and recently completed a series of programmes for a Medical Television channel. In this book he writes in his personal capacity as an experienced general practitioner and senior hospital manager. He is the co-author of *Making Sense of Risk Management*.

Acknowledgements

Helen Kaney, Dento-Legal Adviser at the *St Paul International Insurance Company Ltd.*

Dr Nigel Knott of *DentSure Ltd.*

Dr Mike Mulcahy, formerly of *BUPA DentalCover.*

MAKING THIS BOOK WORK FOR YOU

This is not a read-it-from-cover-to-cover book. Just flip through the pages and get the feel of it.

You will find:

Issues, things that you really should be doing, stuff to think about, a mix of opinion and a cocktail, or two, of conjecture! There are some duplications so that if you dip in and out of the book you can pick up the issues that seem important to you and use them to work on your own, or with colleagues, to go to the heart of the matter, work out your responses and plan for the future.

Coffee breaks! Well, all work and no play – you know what they say! These are located at points in the book where a pause for thought might be a good idea. Don't forget to come back! Take a break, now, and flip through the pages. Not everything will be of use to you. Maybe you already know a thing or two about risk management, or perhaps this is your first attempt to get to grips with it.

Take a break and have a look . . .

Welcome back!

We hope you have come across things in the book that you know already and, hopefully, some things you've never thought of. Perhaps even some stuff to make you think.

When the light comes on there are things to think about. Some are to inform you, give you background and to get you thinking *outside the box* – to look at the issues from a different dimension. Some are deliberately provocative; some just to prove that finding out about serious topics can be fun.

Hazard Warnings are there to point out some tricky issues, or traps not to fall into.

Exercises . . . are there for you to address the issues in the context of where you work and what your task is – regardless of your profession or seniority in the organisation. Use them to get your thinking going and, perhaps, part of your job done. Use them as prompts for team sessions, working together on the challenges that Risk Management brings.

 Make a Note . . . important bits you might want to make a note of . . .

What's in the book? All of these topics are covered:

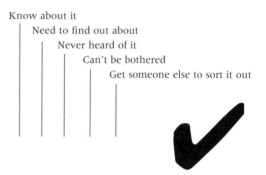

Know about it
　　Need to find out about
　　　　Never heard of it
　　　　　　Can't be bothered
　　　　　　　　Get someone else to sort it out

- What is Risk Management?
- Complaints
- Claims
- Consent
- Confidentiality
- Reviewing the Practice
- The Patients
- The Environment
- Dental Records
- Security of Dental Records
- Patient Access to Dental Records
- Domiciliary Visiting
- Message Taking
- Chaperones
- The Amorous Patient
- Clinical Practice Management
- Standard of Care

Know about it
   Need to find out about
      Never heard of it
         Can't be bothered
            Get someone else to sort it out

- Managing Patient Expectations
- Patient Expectations
- Dental Treatment
- Patient Records
- Radiology
- Children's Radiology
- Dental Caries
- Periodontal Assessment
- Endodontics
- Treatment Planning
- Cosmetic Dentistry
- Dental Laboratories
- Clinical Treatment
- Restorations
- Periodontal Disease
- Broken Instruments
- Crown and Bridge
- Oral Surgery
- Post-Operative Care and Follow-Up
- Prosthetics
- Paedodontics and Orthodontics
- Implants
- Prescriptions and Other Medication
- Managing the Dentist/Patient Relationship
- Health and Safety
- Duties to Staff
- Premises
- Duties to Other Users of Practice Premises
- Employer's Liability
- Enforcement
- First Aid and Collapse Routine
- Fire Safety
- Electricity Regulations

Know about it
  Need to find out about
    Never heard of it
      Can't be bothered
        Get someone else to sort it out

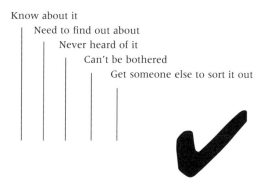

- COSHH Regulations
- Waste Disposal
- Pressure Systems Regulations
- Computers
- Manual Handling
- Medicine Storage
- Pathological Specimens
- Protective Clothing
- Reporting of Injuries, Diseases and Dangerous Occurrences Regulations
- 187
- Cross Infection Control
- Contact with Blood
- Ventilation
- Radiation Hazards
- Care and Maintenance of Dental Equipment
- Finance Management
- Development Plans

Pretty comprehensive, eh? Well worth the money you paid for the book!

WHAT IS RISK MANAGEMENT?

Receiving a complaint from a patient or a solicitor's letter informing you of a patient's intention to sue for an alleged act of negligence is very upsetting. For many dentists, such events are devastating. After trying to provide the best service possible to their patients, to get a *'Dear Sir, on behalf of my client . . .'* in the post is guaranteed to occupy your thoughts and provide some sleepless nights!

The increasingly litigious population, combined with Government and media encouragement to complain has resulted in a spiralling number of patient complaints and claims. One thing's for sure – it'll get worse!

Sorry to be so depressing – but it's time to get real. Risk management is about getting real. Looking at the real risks and addressing them in a real, sensible and methodical way.

Good medical indemnity insurers will encourage you to risk manage your practice and the really good ones will find a way of helping you to do it.

OK, so what is risk management?

Try this:

Risk Management is an insurance and quality control related discipline comprising activities designed to minimise the adverse effects of loss upon a healthcare organisation's human, physical and financial assets through:

- Identification of Loss Potential
- Loss Prevention and Reduction
- Loss Funding and Risk Financing
- Claims Control.

Oh, grim reading! It's the last pompous bit in the book, we promise. Forget that, look at it like this:

1 Identify the risk – establish what is actually likely to go wrong.
2 Analyse the risk – find the chances of something going wrong, its consequences and the potential importance.
3 Control the risk – establish what can be done to reduce, minimise or eliminate it.
4 Cost the risk – calculate the cost of getting it right as opposed to the cost of getting it wrong, i.e. not dealing with it.

One thing's for sure, risk has an impact in all areas of practice:

• clinical activity and awareness of best clinical practice
• the staff
• the premises
• health and safety
• financial assets
• personal risks – reputation and ability to practice.

COMPLAINTS

Let's get this stuff out of the way, right from the start. You're bound to get a complaint sooner or later, so here's how to deal with them with the minimum loss of sleep.

In 1996 a new system for complaints about the NHS replaced the existing system. It was supposed to be better because it:

• gave easy access for complainants
• was simpler than the old system
• separated complaints and disciplinary matters
• made it easier to learn from errors
• created fairness
• provided speedier resolution.

Ho, ho! Ask any dentist who has gone through the grind of an NHS complaint and they will tell you it is, 'cumbersome and difficult'. That is, if they are polite. They are more likely to say, '*&^ %$ ££ ##//>!!!@'!

Here's a quick teach-in on the NHS complaints procedure:

Stages of complaints procedure:

1   Local Resolution including Lay Conciliation (optional)
2   Independent Review
3   Health Service Commissioner (Ombudsman) – not part of the formal
    process.

The Complainant **has the right**:

• to be heard and taken seriously
• to request the assistance of the Community Health Council
• to receive a full explanation of facts and events
• to request an Independent Review
• to complain to the Ombudsman if dissatisfied with the outcome of the
  complaints process.

(The complainant may also complain to the GDC. It used to be a requirement that the complainant swore a statutory declaration of truth when
making a complaint. This is no longer necessary.)

The complainant **has the responsibility**:

• to provide a statement of the complaint
• to explain why if still dissatisfied
• to respond within time scales
• to have respect for the process.

 Make a Note

The complainant **does not have the right**:

• to have an independent review
• to have non-NHS work investigated under the NHS procedure
• to restart the process if still dissatisfied
• to demand any particular action or result.

Timescale: the original complaint must be:

- within six months of the event, or
- within six months of becoming aware of a cause for complaint, provided it is within twelve months of the event.

There is discretion to extend.

Local Resolution. The purpose is to:

- investigate, resolve and/or take action
- respond to complainant as quickly as possible.

The Complaints Manager:

- maintains the timetable
- organises responses
- advises complainant on rights, process and timescale
- makes notes of meetings
- tries to find mutual resolution.

The Lay Conciliator:

- is part of the local resolution process
- **is available to either party**
- reviews correspondence
- speaks to complainant and respondent
- investigates and seeks additional information
- writes full and informative letter to the complainant and respondent.

 Make a Note

Be prepared to work with the conciliator.

Ask for conciliation if the patient is difficult or the complaint is incomprehensible. Co-operation with the conciliator may avoid an independent review at a later stage.

Timescale 2:

- oral complaint – manage on the spot or refer

- acknowledge complaint within two working days or make a full response within five working days (if no acknowledgement)
- full response – ten working days.

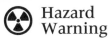 **Hazard Warning**

It's not over when you think it's over . . . complainant can apply for Independent Review within 28 calendar days of receipt of response to Local Resolution.

The Convenor. A lay non-executive member of the health authority (health board in Scotland):

- must act without bias
- considers the issues surrounding an application for an Independent Review
- takes clinical advice on clinical issues
- decides whether Independent Review would **add value** to the resolution.

Lay Chairman. Nominated by the Regional Office on behalf of the Secretary of State:

- advises Convenor
- takes responsibility for the process after Independent Review is accepted
- chairs the Independent Review
- writes and circulates draft and final reports after the Review.

Who sits on an Independent Review panel?

- Chairman
- Convenor
- Lay Member
- Two dental advisers.

What happens?

- complainant and dentist are usually seen separately
- each questioned by panel members
- complainant or dentist may make a statement.

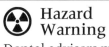 **Hazard**
Warning

Dental advisers may ask questions and advise the panel but take no part in the decision.

After the Independent Review:

- draft report produced by Chairman and sent to dentist and complainant for comment
- final report to CE of health authority
- report sent to dentist and complainant
- CE decides if there is a need for disciplinary action. If so, a Dental Disciplinary Committee Hearing may be convened.

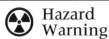 **Hazard**
Warning

Unless you are Perry Mason, (and even if you think you are) never attend an Independent Review alone. You may be accompanied by a friend (LDC representative or defence organisation adviser) but not by a solicitor.

  Dental Disciplinary Hearings are similar to the old-style Dental Service Committees.

Timescale 3:

- if Independent Review is requested, Convenor must acknowledge in two working days
- the Convenor must decide on an Independent Review within ten working days
- if panel agreed, Convenor must make the decision within ten working days
- appointment of panel members within ten working days of decision to create a panel
- draft report within 30 working days of formal appointment of panel
- final report within ten further working days
- report sent out to all parties within five further working days.

The Health Service Commissioner (Ombudsman) may investigate:

- dentist/patient hardship or injustice
- out-of-time decisions
- decision to refuse Independent Review.

Will not investigate:

- on-going complaints
- disciplinary matters
- those complaints where a claim has been instigated.

 Hazard Warning

Cases are selective and the Ombudsman only investigates a small percentage. They may take up to a year to achieve an outcome. The Ombudsman has been known to adopt a name-and-shame policy for dentists who remove patients unreasonably from their lists or who fail to apologise when considered appropriate.

The best tip of all: if you receive a complaint, let your medical indemnity insurers know and they will advise you on the best way to deal with it.

 Make a Note

COMPLAINTS FROM PRIVATE PATIENTS

At present no unified system exists for private patient complaints. For most issues that arise within the practice, the same principles apply as for NHS complaints and a similar system can be employed.

Watch out for the impact of the Human Rights Act. This is new territory and no one really knows how it might impact on complaints procedures. As a rule of thumb the process should be independent, known to both sides in advance, transparent and allow for an appeal.

There is a great book on the topic, published by Radcliffe Medical Press, called *Understanding the Human Rights Act* by, well . . . guess who?

COMPLAINTS CHECKLIST

Get this lot right and you can sleep a bit easier!

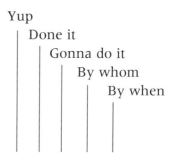

Yup
  Done it
    Gonna do it
      By whom
        By when

- Practice has a system for managing complaints?
- Nominated member of staff to manage the complaints process?
- Timescale for the complaints procedure known to the staff and the dentists?
- Dentists or the complaints manager try to meet any patient who complains to attempt to resolve the problem?
- Details of the complaints procedure published in the Practice Leaflet?
- Details of the complaints procedure displayed on a suitable notice in the waiting area?
- Complaints manager seeks advice about complaints from medical indemnity provider or the LDC?
- If dentist is called to an Independent Review ensure that a dento-legal adviser or an LDC secretary accompanies him.
- Dentist offers an apology if the situation warrants it?
- Practice has policy for refunding payments if the situation warrants it?

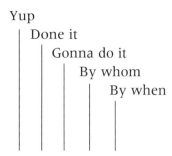

Yup
Done it
Gonna do it
By whom
By when

- Record kept of all complaints?
- Complaints audited and reviewed within
  the practice to decide whether there should
  be action or change and, if so, who should
  be responsible for it?

CLAIMS

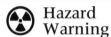 **Hazard Warning**

The risk of a patient making a claim against a dentist is over ten times more likely than it was ten years ago. Currently it is estimated that about one dentist in 30 will be sued by a patient in any given year.

That's just to get your attention! But, it does show how tricky this situation is getting.

However, there is some good news, of all claimant cases:

- three quarters result in no payment to the claimant
- one in five is resolved by negotiation
- only one in 20 gets as far as court.

 Take a break and read this next bit – you need to know it and the fact that you do will impress your colleagues! It's all about the so-called Bolam test. Get up-to-speed on the Bolam test with this quick teach-in.

The test respects the fact that medical opinion is not homogeneous, that there is a range of decisions that may be taken in respect of a single patient, all of which may attract the support of responsible doctors. So, the fact that something has gone wrong does not prove negligence. Medicine cannot guarantee results. In order to win damages, the patient must prove that the error was *negligent*.

The principle of law is:

> *A doctor is not negligent if he has acted in accordance with a practice accepted as proper by a responsible body of medical men skilled in that particular art . . . a doctor is not negligent . . . merely because there is a body of opinion that takes a contrary view* (Bolam v Friern Hospital Mngt Ctte [1957] 2 All ER 118)

Although Bolam related to a medical case, it applies equally to dental issues.

So, what to do if the *'Dear Sir on behalf of my client . . .'* letter from a solicitor turns up in the post, alongside the holiday brochures and the gas bill.

Here's what not to do.

• Don't throw away the solicitor's letter and book a holiday, because if you do they'll cut the gas off!

Here's what you should do.

• Don't panic.
• Don't respond to a solicitor's letter directly, send it to your dental defence company and let them reply – that's what you pay your fees for. And then . . .
• Collect together all relevant notes, correspondence and investigations.
• Do not deface, alter or destroy any of the notes or other records. If you wish to expand previous records for clarification or explanation do so as recommended in Section 7.2 Dental Records.
• Seek an early meeting with your insurer.
• Pay the gas bill.
• Pick a holiday . . .

 Make a Note

Insurers are set up to sort out complaints. They are good at it and that is what you pay the premiums for. They'll love you if you let them know, straight away, that you've got a problem. If you hide the problem then you'll have two problems to deal with, instead of one – the first problem with the patient and the second with the insurers. Insurers understand that even the best dentists and well-run practices will have complaints made about them. They don't see complaints as a black mark – they do see hiding a complaint as original sin!

Here's some other stuff to think about.

- Tell the truth to the person looking after your case, however embarrassing! It gives the best opportunity of achieving the least damaging resolution if they know the full facts.
- Do not let anger cloud your judgement. Stay calm and avoid the red-mist!
- Identify any witnesses that might be able to give evidence for you – practice staff, relatives of the claimant – and give their details to your defence adviser.
- Do not delay in providing required information. Timescales are much tighter under the new Civil Procedure Rules – *see below for an explanation.*

And, be prepared to have a discussion about whether or not to defend or settle the claim. Ouch! Yes, we know it hurts your pride. But let's be practical. The best of us make cock-ups from time to time. Is it time to put your hands in the air and say, 'Oops, sorry . . .'? Think about:

- the view of other experts (flick back to the Bolam pages and think again)
- the likely local damage to reputation through bad publicity
- the intensity of *desire to fight* whatever the consequences
- the fact that you are not the only dentist to suffer a claim. It happens to most dentists at some time.

The Civil Procedure Rules: (as promised)

The 26 April 1999 was a big day for the lawyers and, consequently, the rest of us! The most fundamental reform of the Civil Justice System since the 1870s took effect.

The new Civil Procedure Rules were the result of a long consultative process led by The Rt. Hon. The Lord Woolf, Lord Chief Justice and head-honcho of the law. They are known colloquially as 'The Woolf Reforms'.

The purpose of the reforms was to:

- ensure fairness allowing both parties to be on an even playing field
- minimise or avoid expense

- ensure that cases are dealt with in ways that are proportionate to value, importance and complexity
- ensure that cases are dealt with expeditiously.

Under the new arrangements a case has to follow a number of protocols prior to commencement of legal proceedings. These 'pre-action protocols' place onerous time limits on the dentist.

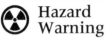 **Hazard**
Warning

If you have a problem contact your insurer. This is all very tricky and the time limits are tight. You may be in more trouble by not moving quickly than from the complaint itself!

A so-called 'letter of claim' is sent by the claimant or solicitor once there is *an intention to sue*. The timetable requires that the claimant provides details before the process commences, including details of the claim, injuries, etc. A letter of acknowledgement **must be sent by the defendant**, that means you, if you are the dentist, but is in reality your dental defence adviser or their appointed legal adviser, **within fourteen days**. See why it is important not to sit on an ugly letter? Make a resolution to send anything like this to your insurers the day you get it – in the lunchtime post!

A letter of response must be sent by the defendant's team within three months of the letter of claim. It must state whether liability is accepted or denied, giving reasons. Copies of all relevant documents must be supplied to the patient. Either party can make an offer to settle.

Three months may sound like a long time but it's not if you take into account getting face to face with people, digging up documents, the state of the postal service and the price of chips . . .

There's more . . .

Experts may be instructed but they must be justified by the party providing the instruction.

If the defendant or the legal adviser does not respond to the claimant in full within three months, the claimant may then commence legal proceedings without fear that the costs will not be allowed on the basis that proceedings have been issued prematurely. So now you see why the insurers want to know what's going on. If there's a delay, they don't hit the timescales and the defence goes pear shaped. They are looking down the twin barrels of costs and costs – and they don't like that!

Make a Note

The Data Protection Act 1998, which came into force on 1 March 2000, entitles a patient to obtain a copy of all computerised and manual records held by the practice.

As with the previous data protection legislation, a copy of the dental records must be provided within 40 days of a request by a patient (or his or her legal representative). A reasonable charge may be made for this.

The Access to Health Records Act 1990 now only applies to requests for disclosure of the dental records of a deceased patient.

CLAIMS CHECKLIST

Get this right and you should be OK . . .

Yup, done it
Ouch, not done it
Will get it done
By whom
By when

- If a dentist is aware of an incident that might give rise to a claim is insurer notified?
- Does the system allow for the earliest possible warning of any claim?
- Does the dentist recognise the potential hazard in an unexpected outcome, e.g. brain damage, unexpected death, physical damage and iatrogenic injury?
- Does the dentist know not to respond directly to a solicitor's letter but to contact the insurer immediately?
- Does the dentist collect together all notes, records, investigations, X-rays and other documents as soon as there is a notification of a possible claim?

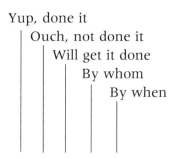

Yup, done it
Ouch, not done it
Will get it done
By whom
By when

- Does the dentist meet with the case handler as soon as possible to plan the management of the case?
- Does the dentist ensure that he tells the case handler the truth no matter how embarrassing?
- Does the dentist keep all correspondence relating to a legal case in a separate file, not in the patient's dental record?
- Are all dentists and staff instructed not to discuss any claim or potential claim with anyone other than a representative of the insurer or lawyer instructed by them?
- Is all evidence of an accident preserved (e.g. needle broken during injection) in case of claim?
- Are immediate copies of records made to avoid any possible allegations of tampering?

CONSENT

Who said you could do that?

Successful relationships between dentists and patients depend on trust and goodwill. When that goes, everything is missing. Preserving the relationship is crucial. However, the balance in the relationship is shifting. The view within the profession is shifting from the dentist providing the amount of information that a 'reasonable dentist' would give in the circumstances (that's the Bolam stuff again – see previous pages), to the dentist having to provide the amount of information that a 'prudent patient' would want to know – from a dentist-centred to a patient-centred emphasis.

Hazard Warning

Patients have the right to decide whether to undergo any dental intervention, even when refusal may result in harm to themselves. Crazy, but there's loadsa case law on this.

Time for a 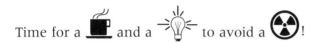 and a ⚡💡⚡ to avoid a ☢!

- Consent may be implied, oral or written.
- A patient who opens his mouth to allow a dentist to do an examination may be assumed to have consented to that examination.
- If a patient consents orally, a note should be added to the patient's record confirming the provision and nature of the consent.
- Written consent is not normally essential or a guarantee but provides a useful document if evidence is required months or years later.
- Consent based on clear explanations is essential, and particularly so in situations such as wisdom tooth extraction, sedation and general anaesthesia.
- The GDC requires written consent for GA and sedation procedures.

And . . .

- Patients must be given sufficient information to enable them to make an informed decision.
- The amount of information depends on a range of factors including the nature of the condition, risks and the patient's wishes.
- Patients may need more information about procedures with high risks or with serious personal, social or professional implications.
- Explanations should be given by a knowledgeable practitioner and ideally by the practitioner carrying out the procedure.
- It may be appropriate for the patient to bring a friend, relative, interpreter, etc.

So . . .

Ensure there is a consent form for any intrusive procedure or any other procedure where a documented record is essential or advisable. Information provided must or may include the following.

- Details of diagnosis and prognosis if the condition is left untreated.
- Uncertainties about diagnosis and options for further investigation prior to treatment.

- Options for management and treatment including the option not to treat.
- Other subsidiary treatments such as pain relief.
- Common and serious side effects.
- Benefits.
- An indication if the process is untested or for research purposes.

And, unless you are Mystic Meg, avoid making assumptions about patients' views. Discuss matters with them and seek information about their concerns. Give the patient a clear explanation of the scope of consent being sought.

- Ensure a system for providing the patient with time (and where appropriate a copy of the consent form). Ideally the patient should discuss the matter with family, friends, etc.
- Ensure that it is understood that 'serious harm' does not mean that the patient would become upset or decide to refuse treatment.
- Ensure that the patient is competent and make a suitable note in the record if you decide that the patient is not competent.

 Make a Note

A dentist should refer to the patient's GP for a psychiatric or psychogeriatric review to assess competence if he or she is unsure whether the patient is competent.

Explanations may be enhanced by using brochures, diagrams, photographs, etc. Remember, what is routine to the dentist is a once in a lifetime experience for most patients. Once authority is obtained it is important not to exceed its scope – except in an emergency.

Consent must not be given under duress, either from family or the practitioner. A patient should be given time to consider the issue before finally consenting. If they say 'no' and they are competent to say 'no' then 'no' it is, no matter how daft it may seem to the dentist.

The practitioner should ensure that the patient is aware of any hazard which might cause the patient concern or to which significance would be attached. Any relevant information withheld from the patient should be recorded together with the reason for doing so. You'd better have a really good reason to withhold information. Usually it is in the area of, 'to provide it would cause the patient serious harm'.

Some patients still hate a trip to the dentist – can't imagine why! Sometimes they don't want to know what you're doing, digging about in their mouth. If a patient declines to know details of their treatment or condition it is still necessary to provide basic information with the option of learning more.

Establishing capacity to make decisions: in legal speak, a person is deemed to have the capacity to make a valid decision to consent or refuse a treatment or other procedure if:

- the issues and information can be understood
- he or she can be believed
- the person can weigh the information in the balance to arrive at a decision.

There's loadsa case-law on this topic and it is a minefield. Common sense is a good guide, if in doubt don't do anything, get a second opinion and above all make really good notes about the decision you arrived at and why.

Remember: no one can provide consent on behalf of an adult, even if the person lacks the capacity to make a decision for him or herself. The existence of diagnosed mental illness does not automatically remove a patient's legal capacity to consent or refuse treatment. Just because a patient is the subject of a compulsory treatment order under a section of the Mental Health Act (1983) (or the Mental Health Act (Scotland) 1984), this does not remove the need to obtain consent for procedures which are unrelated to the mental illness.

 Make a Note

If a patient is not competent to make a decision, the practitioner may provide any investigation or treatment that he or she judges to be in the patient's best interests.

What about the kids then? Mmm . . . tricky this and getting trickier!

Children under 16 may be able to consent to investigations or treatment if they understand the nature, purpose and possible consequences of the proposed treatment and the consequences of non-treatment. They must not suffer duress from family or friend.

Here's a quick teach-in on some stuff you should know about – even if it is only to show off!

Rights of 'Gillick' Competent Children

Remember Mrs Gillick? Her daughter wanted to go on the pill. The Doc' said OK. Mum didn't know anything about it, and thought she should have been consulted about the matter. The roof came in and case law was made!

A child is 'Gillick' competent when he or she has sufficient maturity and understanding to consent to the treatment in question. Obviously, children may be capable of comprehending some treatments but not others and not all children develop at the same rate. Children must understand the risks, benefits and consequences of non-treatment and must not make a decision under duress.

However, so long as they are competent with respect to the *particular* procedure proposed, they too are entitled to information and the right to consent to it.

Here's the important bit: 'they are competent with respect to the *particular* procedure proposed'. Remember the recent case where a teenager didn't want heart surgery because she thought the process was too overwhelming and didn't want a life-time of dependency on pills and treatment? The court decided it was good for her and doctors might have been in the difficult situation where they could have forced treatment on a patient who didn't want it. In the end they were let off the hook because the teenager changed her mind and consented to treatment. Phew! Close shave for the Docs.

However, the approach to children is not identical to adults. Adults have the right to consent to, *or refuse* treatment. 'Gillick' competent children have the right to consent, but their right to refuse is more restricted.

The logic for this is that, with children, parents also retain rights to consent on their behalf. So even though a child may refuse treatment, lawful consent may be supplied by a parent.

This happened in *Re W (a minor): Medical treatment* [1992] 4 All ER 627. A sixteen-year-old girl suffered from a serious eating disorder and was at risk of suffering serious harm. She refused her consent to treatment. Her parents both consented. The Court of Appeal ordered treatment to take place in her 'best interests'.

Got all that! What does it mean for the dentist? Well, the short answer, it means the same for the dentist as it does the doctor. Treatment without consent is permitted in certain circumstances (principally life-threatening emergencies). These are highly unlikely ever to arise in dental practice and should, in any case, be confined to the minimum intervention necessary to save life or to prevent an irrevocable deterioration in the patient's condition.

Pleased you became a dentist and not a doctor?

CONSENT CHECKLIST

Get this right and you should be OK . . .

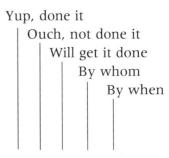

Yup, done it
Ouch, not done it
Will get it done
By whom
By when

- Do the dentists and staff understand the concept of consent?
- Do the dentists obtain consent for any procedure which might be considered intrusive by the patient?
- Does the dentist seek written consent for more complex or intrusive procedures?
- Does the dentist understand that a refusal to consent to a procedure that would or might be beneficial is the patient's right?
- Does the dentist always obtain the patient's consent before supplying information to a third party?
- Does the dentist ensure that there is a signed consent for any post-marketing surveillance or research?
- If the patient does not sign a consent form does the dentist record consent in the dental record?
- Does the consent take note of the nature of the contract, i.e. NHS or private, and ensure that the patient is consenting to the appropriate treatment?
- Does the consent include an estimate of cost?

CONFIDENTIALITY

An ethical requirement of all dentists, confidentiality is the cornerstone of good practice. Patients have the right to expect that information learned during the course of professional duties will not be disclosed. Such confidential information should be protected from improper disclosure when disposed of, stored, transmitted or received. The patient has the freedom to decide which personal information should be made public or semi-public.

If information is not kept confidential:

- patients may be reluctant to, or may refuse to, disclose any information
- inadequate information may impede sound diagnosis or management
- patients may refuse to attend at all

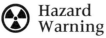 **Hazard Warning**

All practitioners and employees have a common law and professional duty to protect the confidentiality of the patient.

The Caldicot review of Patient Identifiable Information recommended that NHS organisations should be held accountable through clinical governance procedures for continuously improving confidentiality and security procedures governing the access and storage of personal information.

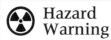 **Hazard Warning**

When documents are destroyed they must be incinerated or shredded with appropriate safeguards for confidentiality throughout the procedure.

It's not just you – it's the others as well . . .

Dentists are responsible for breaches of confidentiality by those staff that they employ. Essentially **all** information should be kept confidential.

There are some exceptions.

- In the public interest, e.g. to avoid someone being exposed to serious harm or death.
- Where the duty of care to an individual overrides the duty of confidentiality to another.

These circumstances virtually never occur in the context of a dental practice. Or do they? Perhaps you know better!

 Make a Note

What happens when the Old Bill turns up and want to look at 'chummies dental records, guv, 'cos 'e's bitten a bloke's ear off in the pub'?

The police:

- do **not** have access to dental records
- do **not** have access to appointment books.

The answer is, 'sorry officer'. You see, if the police require information they should seek a judicial order under *The Police and Criminal Evidence Act 1984*, or through a court order in Scotland.

If you get a confidentiality issue wrong the consequences are likely to be:

- a complaint to the practice
- a complaint to the GDC – it could be serious professional misconduct
- a civil action.

This may lead to:

- damage to personal relationships
- damage to the business
- . . . and a shed load of publicity you can do without.

So please try to get this one right.

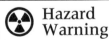 **Hazard Warning**

If a health authority is aware of an incident involving a breach of confidentiality it may itself refer the matter to the GDC or direct the patient to make a complaint.

Make a Note

Overall it is usually easier to defend a *failure to inform* than it is to defend an inappropriate breach of information.

There's nothing like gossip!

The Dental Practice environment is a key area where confidentiality may be breached. Casually made telephone calls that may involve the release of patient information, conversations with patients in environments which lend themselves to being overheard and gossip may all result in breaches of confidentiality. Check the telephone environment – is it easy to overhear what's being said?

CONFIDENTIALITY CHECKLIST

Get this right and you must be nearly there!

> Yup, it's OK
> > Ouch, no
> > > Will get it sorted
> > > > By whom
> > > > > By when

- Do the reception staff understand the importance of confidentiality?
- Do the reception staff understand that a breach of confidentiality may result in a disciplinary procedure and could lead to instant dismissal?
- Is it possible to overhear telephone conversations in the reception area?
- Is there a part of the reception where a patient can speak in confidence without being overheard?

REVIEWING THE PRACTICE

What's it like over at your place?

The only way to find out is to do a risk management audit. Sounds difficult? No, easy stuff. The idea is to spot what is likely to screw up and then do something about it. There are several approaches.

You could hire in an expensive herd of management guru types who would do it for you – and charge so much you'll never be able to afford to eat meat again.

You could ask for the help of your dental defence insurers. They like to know that you're running a tight ship. That way they expect to get less claims.

And, you could sort this out yourself. Here's how . . .

EIGHT STEPS FOR IMPLEMENTING A RISK MANAGEMENT SYSTEM

1 **Identify key risk areas**. The trick here, is to involve everyone. Use brain-storming techniques and interviews with staff to get their views on where the risks are. Take time to review past incidents, check previous claims and complaint histories and talk with patients.

2 **Identify key trigger events**. Look for trends. History is the great foreteller of the future. If it's happened before, what's to stop it happening again? Keep an eye out for national incidents – could it happen to you?

3 **Implement an incident reporting system**. There is no great sin in getting something wrong. The best of well run organisations make a mess of it at some stage or other. The sin is not knowing something has gone wrong, or having the incident covered up. Much has been said and written about the so-called 'whistle-blowing' policies in the NHS. It's daft to call something as important as this 'whistle-blowing'. Who wants to blow the whistle? Makes you sound like a referee at the big match. Encourage the kind of atmosphere in the practice that, if someone does make a mistake, they feel OK about letting people know. British Airways are very good at this. They have a senior captain (nick-named The Pope), who staff can confess foul-ups, glitches and mistakes to without the fear of being bawled out, or given the sack. Encourage a no blame culture. Be sure to cultivate an atmosphere where staff feel able to talk about a 'near-

miss'. It is good to learn from our mistakes but even better to learn from other people's. However, to learn we must know about them.

4 **Investigate high risk events.** When something does go wrong, investigate it immediately, even if all the facts are not immediately to hand. Look into what happened, get a feel for the likely causes and make sure you act quickly to avoid a recurrence, even if it means you put temporary restrictions and policies in place. Better to move first and change back later than have something bad go wrong, again. Take care when obtaining statements from staff. They may be nervous, cautious and feel under threat. Create an atmosphere where they feel relaxed about being frank. Consider support networks for staff and those involved.

5 **Monitor and analyse reports for trends.** Buy an anorak and be a trend-spotter. Risk management is all about trying to predict what might go wrong and the best indicators are likely to be trends. Track complaints, minor injuries, accidents – regularly. They will give you a clue to the bigger picture. Be honest about events and don't be tempted to fudge unpleasant truths. And, don't rush to judgement! If you can do all that, forget the anorak, just wear your underpants over your trousers and jump tall buildings in a single stride!

6 **Implement changes in practice as necessary.** No point having all this trend analysis stuff if you're not going to make use of it. Beware, even where obvious change is called for, it will still have to be 'managed into the practice'. This is true of both clinical practice and managerial practice. Start by ensuring everyone understands the reason for change. Even if they don't agree, make sure they understand the motives behind it.

7 **Education and feedback.** Folk generally don't come to work intent on fouling up. They often do it out of ignorance. Be sure there are regular feedback opportunities and, where necessary, staff training and education initiated so that risks in the future can be avoided.

8 **Consider an outside company with expertise in risk management.** You cannot expect to have all the answers, but you can be expected to know where to go to find them. Start by networking with other practices. Have they had the same problems? Compare your problems and share your solutions. Use a guru, but watch the costs.

Other sources of help may include:

- the health authority
- the Local Dental Committee
- the Primary Care Group (or LHCC in Scotland)

- commercial organisations such as pharmaceutical and insurance companies
- the Faculty of General Dental Practitioners, the Royal College of Surgeons.

Try this simple ranking system to get a feel for the size of the problem:

$$\text{Risk} = \frac{\text{Likelihood}}{\text{of}} \times \frac{\text{Severity}}{\text{of}}$$
$$\text{Hazard} \qquad \text{Consequences}$$

Risk factor = Numerical Representation of Risk

Where one is low and five is high, take a number between one and five to express the likelihood of the hazard and the same for the severity of the consequences. Multiply them together and use that as a numerical expression of relative risk.

WHO'S THE RISKY PERSON?

Appoint someone in the practice to be the risk management lead. Here's a basic outline of what you can expect them to deliver.

For each part of the practice:

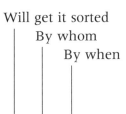

Will get it sorted
    By whom
        By when

- define the hazard – use brainstorming, analysis of any data, information from service users
- define the potential risk sufferer – the clinician, the practice, the staff or the patient, carer or family
- identify existing controls
- identify requirements to achieve improvement

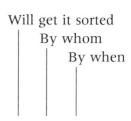

Will get it sorted
By whom
By when

- identify who in the practice can take the responsibility for achieving the change – can it be a part of the normal day, do they have the skills, do they need training, what are the financial implications?
- set realistic targets for improvement
- record progress
- measure outcomes by audit and peer review.

PRACTICE REVIEW CHECKLIST

Do this and you are on your way . . .

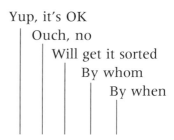

Yup, it's OK
Ouch, no
Will get it sorted
By whom
By when

- Are there arrangements in place for the practice team to develop their own checklist for reviewing the practice?
- Is there a system in place for reviewing the practice for risk?
- Is there a mechanism for staff to report 'near misses'?
- Is there a mechanism for patients to pass suggestions to the practice (e.g. through a suggestion box)?
- Is there a staff member to identify, implement and co-ordinate any risk reduction procedures in the practice?

THE ENVIRONMENT

No, not the hole in the ozone layer just above the surgery. This is about the surgery. It's cost a lot of money to build and maintain and it's worth looking after even if only for the sake of making sure it continues to make a substantial investment in someone's pension fund. More impor- tantly, the public are in and out of the place and staff work there. Consequently, it must be safe for the public and meet all the require- ments of health and safety. *(There's more on Health and Safety later in the Tool Kit).*

The surgery should be thoroughly inspected by a team of staff, including one or more of the dentists, the practice manager, a dental nurse and one or more senior receptionists. The assessment should be done from the perspective of the patient, both adult and child. Each area should be examined in turn and any risks identified, analysed and solutions sought.

Here's a list of the type of things they should be looking for:

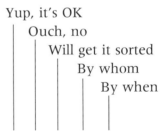

Yup, it's OK
Ouch, no
Will get it sorted
By whom
By when

The Reception/Waiting Area:

- Is the entrance door easy for a patient to open?
- Is there a disabled access?
- Is the reception on one level?
- If doors are fully glazed are there markings to indicate the presence of glass for a partially sighted patient?
- Is glass in doors toughened or laminated?
- Is there a part of the reception desk at a suitable height for patients in wheelchairs?

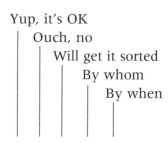

Yup, it's OK
  Ouch, no
    Will get it sorted
      By whom
        By when

- Is there a hearing loop for deaf patients?
- Is there an area where a patient can speak in confidence to a receptionist?
- Is the telephone situated such that patients waiting in reception cannot hear conversations with patients?
- Is the telephone system adequate for the number of calls received?
- Are there sufficient chairs?
- Are patients kept informed of delays in being seen?
- Are there adequate instructions about what to do if not called within an agreed time?
- Are all parts of the waiting area visible to staff?
- Is the area adequately heated and ventilated?
- Are carpets of good quality (not frayed) and suitably fitted to minimise the risk of a patient tripping?
- Are floors safe and not slippery?
- Is there a notification about complaints, concerns and compliments?

Toilets:

- Do they meet requirements for disabled patients?
- Is there an alarm for a patient unwell in the toilet?
- Can the door to the toilet be opened by a staff member from the outside?

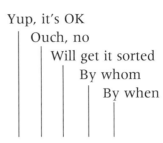

Yup, it's OK
Ouch, no
Will get it sorted
By whom
By when

Consulting/Treatment Rooms:

- Is the dental surgery of adequate size, heated, lit and ventilated?
- Is the dental chair appropriately located and is the dental light in the correct position for maximum illumination?
- Is the sharps box inaccessible to small children?
- Are instruments, syringes, etc. kept securely?
- Are prescription pads and other documents kept secure?
- Is the room equipped with a panic alarm?
- Are there secure facilities for infected and other hazardous waste?
- Is the floor safe?

General:

- Is the lighting adequate?
- Is the décor of suitable colours for partially sighted patients?
- Do doors open safely?

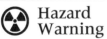 **Hazard Warning**

The standards expected of surgeries are rising. It is a good idea to inspect the whole building on a regular basis to ensure that standards are met.

PRACTICE ENVIRONMENT CHECKLIST

Just when you thought you'd done it all – just to be sure . . .

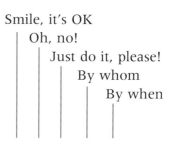

Smile, it's OK
Oh, no!
Just do it, please!
By whom
By when

- Does the practice have a disabled access?
- Does the practice have a part of the reception area accessible to patients in wheelchairs?
- Does the practice have a hearing loop?
- Can a patient speak privately to a receptionist in the reception area?
- Can the patients read any information about other patients recorded in appointment books, message books or dental records?
- Are any VDU screens in the reception area that may show patient information visible to other patients in the reception area?
- Can patients overhear information about other patients?
- Are there disabled toilet facilities?
- Are there adequate toilets for male and female patients and staff?
- Is there an effective appointment system which has the flexibility to meet the needs of patients with emergencies.
- Can a patient obtain an urgent appointment quickly?
- Are patients notified if the dentist is running late?
- If a dentist is running late can the patient be offered an appointment with an alternative dentist if appropriate?

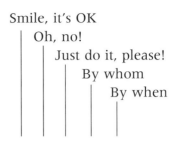

Smile, it's OK
Oh, no!
Just do it, please!
By whom
By when

- Does the practice display any appointment targets, e.g. maximum waiting time to obtain an appointment?
- Are the practice telephone numbers clearly displayed in the practice leaflet and in the waiting area?
- Are the receptionists given clear instructions about how to manage an urgent call received at reception?
- Is the reception notice board regularly inspected and obsolete notices removed?
- Are there adequate telephone lines for the practice?
- Are the receptionists trained in interpersonal skills?
- Is communication good between staff members?
- Does the practice comply with the Patient's Charter requirements?
- Is the practice developing protocols for use by receptionists?

DENTAL RECORDS

What's your favourite record? Paul Lambden likes anything by Des O'Connor. Roy Lilley prefers Max Bygraves!

We all know the jokes about doctors' handwriting. No doubt the same is true of dentists! True or not, times are changing and a higher standard of record keeping is becoming par for the course.

Here are just a few of the changes that can impact on record keeping.

- The greater involvement of patients in making choices about their own dental care.

- Patients' access to their own records.
- The increasing use of computers.
- Clinical audit and governance.

What constitutes 'records'. Well, the rules say records should contain the famous five:

- Identify the patient.
- Support the diagnosis.
- Justify the treatment.
- Document the course and results.
- Promote the continuity of care among healthcare providers.

Clinical records do not have to show that the patient went home with a beautiful smile. They just have to show that the dentist acted reasonably, according to accepted standards, regardless of the outcome . . .

 Make a Note

The Data Protection Act came into force in March 2000. It replaced the provisions of the Access to Health Records Act 1990 and gives access to the patient to all dental records including all electronic records. The legislation is in force in all parts of the United Kingdom.

By the way, records are supposed to be complete, legible and accurate. The complete and accurate bit doesn't seem to be a problem, it's the legible bit we seem to have most trouble with! *(More later!)*

What else about records? Well, here are five more things they are supposed to do.

- Meet legal and service requirements.
- Provide information and communication between practitioners.
- Document the care as a basis for planning care and treatment.
- Allow for the evaluation and progress of the patient.
- Change therapies where effectiveness has not been demonstrated.

Let's get risky.

Now we know the rules, what are some of the potential risks that we need to manage? Here are a few ideas, to get the juices flowing:

Problem	Solution
Identify the patient without risk of error – look out for two patients with identical or very similar names.	Make sure the notes have a *name hazard* sticker on them.
Ensure the continuity of care.	Accurate and contemporary notes, comprehensive.
Enable communication between practitioners.	Clear data on what has been prescribed and done, the responses to treatment and a demonstration as to how clinical decisions have been arrived at.
Allow for concurrent or retrospective review.	Chronological records of a sequence of events, the factors observed and the response to treatment.
Allow for the collection of data for research/educational purposes.	Clarity of all elements.
Sufficient information to protect the dentist and the patient.	Allow for patients to examine their own records and be involved in their care through informed consent. Research shows where patients have made a complaint and been shown their records, they are less likely to pursue a complaint if the records are complete and clear. Where they are scant and indecipherable the patient is more likely to become suspicious and pursue the complaint.

Nothing else could go wrong with documentation, could it?

You wanna bet! Take a look at this lot!

LEGIBILITY

It's not too much to ask, is it? Why can't practitioners write nicely? They say docs write badly so they can get off the hook – they write a squiggle and pretend it means anything. The trouble is, it might mean 'anything' to a fellow dentist seeing the same patient and trying to work off the notes.

The patient has a perfect right to see his or her dental record and also has an entitlement to understand it. The dentist may be called upon to explain the meaning of notes made. Misinterpreting a set of notes can be disastrous. Hypertension can easily be muddled up with hypotension. See what I mean?

 Make a Note

A great trick some barristers play is to ask a dentist to read an entry he or she wrote, perhaps years earlier. If it cannot be read, the dentist looks really stupid – and dangerous. Ouch!

Exercise

Describe how you would arrange to sample dental records for legibility. Consider issues such as patient confidentiality.

Also, how would you approach a colleague suffering from *chronic-handwriting-unreadability-itis?*

BLANK SPACES

This is a great trick. A few well chosen spaces can be left and filled in at a later date. It has been known to work quite well. The problem is, these days, ink can be forensically dated. Mmmm, embarrassing if a word or sentence in the middle of the notes can be shown to be three years younger than its parent paragraph! Do you like porridge? I think they still serve it in prison, don't they?

ALTERATIONS TO THE RECORD

Never destroy, or rewrite a previous record, tempting though it may be. In the past it might have been possible to get away with it. The problem is, these days patients have access to their records. If they turn up in court with a copy of their records, which look nothing like the copy you have brought along from the practice – well, it's back to the porridge for someone!

ARE WE LABOURING THE POINT ABOUT GOOD RECORDS?

Yes, without an apology. Here's a repeat of the reason. Cut it out and stick it on the surgery fridge with one of those magnet thingys, or tape it to your forehead:

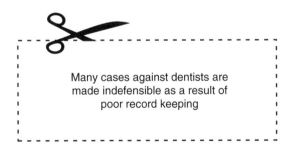

Many cases against dentists are made indefensible as a result of poor record keeping

Here's the gold standard. The dentist should ensure:

- consistency of reporting and recording
- consistency of record organisation

- consistency of management of the records in respect of completing FP17s (GP17s in Scotland) and organising recall systems
- confidentiality
- quality assurance
- access to information through appropriate recording, clear handwriting and avoidance of the use of unfamiliar abbreviations
- that records are made contemporaneously or as nearly contemporaneously as possible. Writing up records once a significant time has elapsed, brings with it the risk that important facts may be omitted. This could have serious consequences.
- that care is taken that there is no risk of confusing two patients with the same or similar names. If a patient has a common name, e.g. Smith, the notes should carry with them a warning to check the address or date of birth of the patient at the time of the consultation to ensure that the correct notes have been selected. It is also helpful to spell out complex names phonetically to ensure that they can be pronounced correctly during any patient encounter. To mispronounce a patient's name may often set a consultation off on the wrong foot and may be offensive.
- that record entries are made only by those people who are authorised to do so. In general, this will be the dentist, the dental surgery assistants, hygienist and nurse practitioners. Anyone entering information on the record should have a consistent style.

Isn't all this a bit of a fag?

Many dentists feel that to record all relevant information places a large burden upon them in terms of the time required. It is important to understand that notes are comprehensive if they include all *relevant* data and it may not be necessary to write large volumes. War and peace is not required. However, dentists should certainly be sensitive to any possibility of a treatment or condition where there is a chance that a patient may end up dissatisfied or frustrated at the end of treatment. In such cases, it is particularly important to record the events surrounding the consultation.

Make a Note

Here's a neat trick

An easy shorthand for managing emergency consultations is to use the SOAP formula. No, not Coronation Street, although it's been around just as long, if not longer! It is used to group the examination and management under four main headings:

- **Subjective**: the patient's own complaints
- **Objective**: the dentist's assessment of the problem
- **Assessment**: the differential diagnosis of the symptoms
- **Plan**: for management and this should be followed by the treatment actually provided.

In assessing what is relevant in the dental record, it is useful to follow a simple rule of thumb. So, in a patient who had not been seen for many years and about whom the dentist had forgotten, from the information in the record it should be possible to:

- establish the clinical state, treatment required and what treatment was provided, when and why
- perform whatever treatment is due for the patient and know why that treatment is necessary.

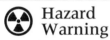 **Hazard Warning**

The dentist is responsible for the acts and omissions of his staff including information documented in the dental record. It is therefore important that the dentist makes explicit what information he does and does not require to be noted down for the avoidance of any confusion.

All records should be legible and signed by the person who made them.

The dentist should regularly check entries made by other staff members to ensure their quality and accuracy. In the event of a complaint or claim arising weeks or months after the event, it will probably be impossible to establish if information written contemporaneously was incomplete or inaccurate.

The record should also include details of any failed appointments.

> ### ☢ Hazard
> ### Warning
>
> One of the biggest problems with dental records occurs when litigation arises and it is not possible to substantiate diagnosis, treatment plan, treatment provided or referral details if they are not supported by appropriate note entries. It is a fundamental requirement that all notes are adequately maintained and therefore a dentist's credibility is seriously diminished if he or she cannot provide documentation to support what has been done.
>
> The measure of the quality of dentist's notes is the good old Bolam test *(see previous references)*. The court will ask what records a reasonable dentist would have kept.
>
> Not only should all routine visits be recorded but every unscheduled or emergency attendance should be noted. It may be particularly important to detail emergency treatment provided because it may be that it is the first sign of a complication or failed treatment and evidence that it was promptly and appropriately managed may be vital in defending the dentist's position.

RECORD QUALITY ASSURANCE

With the development of clinical governance for all doctors and dentists, it is becoming increasingly important that the dentist ensures that his dental records meet quality assurance parameters.

How do you do that? Here's a neat trick . . .

Pick out, at random, (say) 20 records per month and inspect them to check that the information documented is accurate and appropriate and reflects the care actually provided for the patient. This is a very good way to pick up trends in mistakes and that is a good pointer to finding out what needs to be changed and often helps to identify the training needs of staff and colleagues. Be sure to keep a record of the checks as they will form part of the evidence of personal and professional development and maintaining standards.

What to look out for when checking the records?

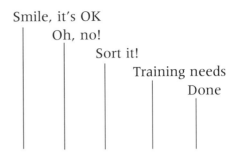

Smile, it's OK
Oh, no!
Sort it!
Training needs
Done

- Is the record appropriately stored, clean and dry?
- Does the record contain adequate information about the patient's medical history and any medication?
- Does the record contain adequate information about the patient's dental status and any significant diagnostic information?
- Does the record contain information about treatment undertaken and materials employed? Is the dosage and type of local anaesthetic recorded?
- Does the record contain information about any referrals made, to whom they were made and the reasons for making such referrals?
- In the case of private patients and in those patients with insurance plans, does the record contain adequate financial information to enable an assessment of probity if required?
- Are entries legible, signed and dated?
- If abbreviations are used, are they clearly understandable? No jokes or pejorative terms?

Make a Note

Never alter contemporaneous records at a later date. If you need to clarify something, or add a detail, do this:

- add an additional card
- date it with the current date
- explain why the additional record is being added, i.e. for clarification, etc.
- write the additional note and file
- do not write notes in pencil

 Hazard Warning

In the event of a claim or a criticism, notes can help you swim, or can sink you. If notes are not clear you'll be in trouble if you need to fish them out and refer to them five years from now. Yes, it does happen. If you can't read your notes, the judge will have a go, prosecuting council will have a go and the press will have a field day.

 Make a Note

For private records it is advisable to retain, store or destroy them using the same criteria as for NHS records.

Here's how:

General Dental Council guidance requires that dental records are stored 'carefully'. There's no definition of 'carefully' but there are some guidelines. The responsibility of the dentist extends to storage, disposal, transfer and destruction of records.

- Current records must be stored on the surgery premises.
- They must be protected from fire, flood and damp.
- Records for patients no longer receiving treatment by the practice must be securely retained.

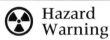 **Hazard Warning**

Any record documents to be destroyed should be incinerated or shredded with appropriate safeguards for confidentiality during the procedure. So, make sure that the *Friend of the Stars*, Benny the Bin-man, can't rummage through your dustbin. This is particularly important for dentists who have well known personalities as patients.

Thinking about up-dating your computer or sending one off for repair? Read this next bit with care.

> Dentists wishing to dispose of computer hardware should ensure that there is no information on the hard disk that can be retrieved. This is particularly important when computers are being sold or when they are being repaired at other premises. The dentist should be sure, either that the hard disk is fully erased. Alternatively they must ensure that the computer and its hard disk have been destroyed before allowing them to be removed to a refuse tip or for other disposal. In the case of repair, the dentist should take steps to prevent the information on the hard disk becoming available to maintenance staff.

 Make a Note

So, now you know – looks like time you found out about back-up onto tape, Zip-files or writeable CDs. In the dark? Try your average 15-year-old!

PATIENT ACCESS TO DENTAL RECORDS

Oops, this is getting a bit tricky. Now you can see why those naughty little *aide-mémoires* about patients could catch you out.

The Data Protection Act 1998 came into force in March 2000. The Act now covers all health records including all electronic records and permits access to all health records whenever they were made. The Act is in force in all parts of the United Kingdom.

Read this bit again:

The Data Protection Act 1998 came into force in March 2000. **The Act now includes all health records** including all electronic records **and permits** access to all health records whenever they were made. The Act is in force in all parts of the United Kingdom.

Get the picture? Old records made 20 years ago on the Isle of Skye still count!

What's a health record? Here's the official version:

> A health record is defined as any record relating to the physical or mental health or condition of an individual and which has been made by a health professional. This may include electronic data, manual data, sound recordings and video recordings.

What happens when a patient asks for a copy of their records? Section 7 of the Data Protection Act says:

- a request must be received in writing and with the appropriate fee
- access should be provided within 40 days and the patient is entitled to receive a copy of the record
- the standard fee payable is £10 for electronic records and a maximum fee of up to £50 for paper records (this may be about to change restricting the maximum fee to £10 for all records).

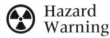 **Hazard Warning**

A patient may request that inaccurate information in the dental record may be corrected. If dissatisfied he or she may complain to the Data Protection Commissioner or apply to the courts for a certificate of compliance.

The court may order a dentist to rectify, erase or destroy inaccurate data or require that the records are supplemented with a statement setting out the true facts.

 Make a Note

All records are now *disclosable* and the previous deadline of 1 November 1991 under the Access to Health Records Act 1990 no longer applies except in respect of deceased patients.

Information that breaches confidentiality of, or relates to, a third party (who is not a health professional) who has not consented to disclosure, may be withheld.

Disclosure may also be withheld if it would be likely to cause serious harm to the physical or mental health or condition of the data subject (patient) or any other person.

Hazard Warning

Just to cheer you up . . . Data subjects (patients) now have a right to claim compensation for damage or distress caused by a breach of the Act.

 Time for a brew – or something stronger! Whilst you check the check-list . . .

DENTAL RECORDS CHECKLIST

Here we go . . .

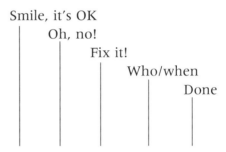

Smile, it's OK
Oh, no!
Fix it!
Who/when
Done

- Are the dental records kept securely?
- Is a system in place for the collection, maintenance, storage, retrieval and distribution of dental records?
- Is a member or members of staff responsible for the confidentiality, security and physical safety of dental records?
- Are dental records maintained in a specific order for easy retrieval of information?
- Is each dental record labelled with the patient's name, NHS number, date of birth, address and registered doctor?
- Is access to dental records appropriate?

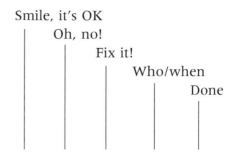

Smile, it's OK
Oh, no!
Fix it!
Who/when
Done

- Do the reception staff understand the *Data Protection Act 1998*?
- Are dental records suitably marked with hazard stickers for patients with similar names?
- Do the notes indicate a patient who may be medically compromised, e.g. taking the drug Warfarin?
- Is there a tracking system for knowing when a dental record is with an individual dentist?
- Is the writing in the record legible?
- Is there a system for arranging the release of patient information? Does this include a written authorisation signed by the parent or guardian where appropriate?
- Is there a procedure for information requiring special release (e.g. HIV, psychiatric detail, alcohol/drugs)?
- Is there a policy for the release of information to a third party?
- Is there a policy for making any charges for the reproduction of dental records?
- Is the dental surgery assistant adequately tutored in dental charting when assisting the dentist?
- Is there a system in place for arranging the removal and storage (if appropriate) of inactive records?
- Are the notes in chronological order?

There's more . . .

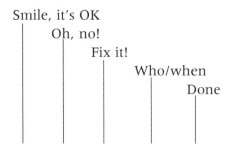

Smile, it's OK
Oh, no!
Fix it!
Who/when
Done

- Are dental records of a suitable quality and sufficiently detailed to be understood at a later date?
- Are notes made contemporaneously?
- Do the dentists avoid the use of abbreviations that are not approved?
- Do the dentists avoid the use of disparaging or pejorative terms in the records?
- Does everyone understand that dental records should never be altered at any time after the consultation?
- Are new patient medical history details entered in the dental record when the patient is first seen?
- Do healthcare professionals other than the dentist enter their own notes in the medical record?
- Are errors in dental records deleted by drawing a single line through the note?
- Are corrections clearly recorded, dated and signed by the author?
- When a patient is referred for a further opinion is there a maximum time agreed for the referral letter to be completed and sent?
- Are computer records kept securely and backed up?
- Is the computer kept securely to minimise the risk of theft or damage?

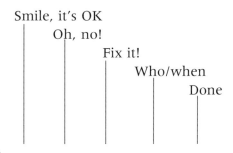

Smile, it's OK
　　Oh, no!
　　　　　Fix it!
　　　　　　　Who/when
　　　　　　　　　　Done

- Is the computer registration with the Data Protection Registry correct and up to date?
- Are arrangements in place to manage requests from patients to amend or erase information in the dental record?
- Is there an effective system to ensure that dentists review all communications and reports before filing?
- Does the dentist initial and date stamp every communication before filing?

 How did you make out? Time for something stronger?

DOMICILIARY VISITING

To go, or not to go? That is the question.

Here are the rules:

> An NHS dentist under his Terms of Service shall visit and treat a patient, whose condition so requires, at the place at which the patient normally resides or is temporarily resident, provided it is not more than twenty miles from the practice premises.

> ## Make a Note
>
> A dentist who provides services privately may make whatever visiting arrangements he or she wishes with any patient who cannot attend the surgery.

Private or not, the same standards of care and treatment are expected whether they are provided in the practice or in a domiciliary visit.

VISIT CHECKLIST

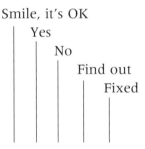

- Does the dentist provide a domiciliary visiting service?
- Does the dentist, if working under the terms and conditions of the NHS, understand the rules concerning mileage incurred when multiple visits are undertaken?
- Does the dentist understand that a lower standard is not acceptable because the patient is not seen in the surgery?
- Does the dentist make arrangements to have a chaperone present whenever appropriate?

MESSAGE TAKING

Message taking? What's that got to do with risk management?

Well, strictly speaking, nothing, something, everything, zilcho and a hell of a lot. Look at it this way. The receptionist is the front-of-house, shop window, first port of call, scene setter and fixer. If the receptionist is pleasant, efficient and on top of the job, a lot of potential problems fly out of the window. If they are rude, flustered, badly trained then appointments get screwed up, messages muddled up and the whole thing becomes a foul-up. A busy practice may receive thirty or more calls an hour and it is essential that any information received for onward transmission to a dentist is taken accurately and reliably and appropriately recorded. Here are a few simple rules and training tips to make a patient's first contact with the surgery a delight. It then allows just the dentist to make a mess of things!

Receptionists, please, when speaking to a patient on the telephone:

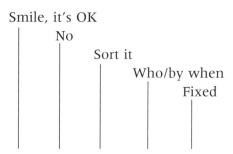

Check!

- identify yourself
- make notes of date and time of call and all relevant information in the message book
- make sure that the call recipient signs each entry
- if the message is taken by the receptionist ensure that the message is passed to the dentist, either immediately if it is urgent or at the first possible opportunity
- ensure that the dentist confirms receipt of the message by signature in the message book.

Thank you!

MESSAGE TAKING CHECKLIST

Get this right and you should be OK. Get the message?

Smile, it's OK
    No
        Sort it
            Who/by when
                Fixed

- Does the practice have a message book?
- Do the receptionists enter messages according to a protocol, i.e. name, address, telephone number and message synopsis?
- Does the dentist sign the message book when a message is collected?

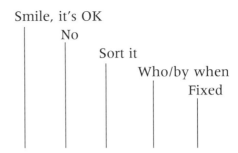

- Do receptionists have authority to give patients information about themselves over the telephone?
- Is there a policy and do receptionists understand that information should only be given out to the patient to whom it relates and not to a third party or left on an answering machine?
- Are all staff aware that an acknowledgement or recognition to a third party that a person is a patient is a breach of confidentiality?

CHAPERONES

Do we have to spell it out?

Some dentists have been accused of some 'embarrassing' behaviour. The dentist works in close proximity to the patient and there is opportunity for actions by either party to be misinterpreted by the other during examination or treatment. Usually the nurse works in the consulting room but, with a risky patient, what happens if the nurse goes out to develop the X-rays?

Be sure to get this right.

- Ensure a chaperone is present during treatment.
- The chaperone may be a member of staff or a relative but, in the latter case, make sure that the relative is present with the patient's consent.
- The dentist should never make suggestive comments to a patient during treatment.
- Some sedative agents have hallucinogenic properties and may generate sexual fantasies. It is vital that a member of the practice staff is present

during the whole of treatment under sedation of any sort to act as
witness and chaperone.

- The dentist should never rest or leave instruments on the chest of a
  patient during treatment.
- Risks are greater out-of-hours when treatment is provided by a dentist
  for a patient with an emergency. The dentist should take steps to ensure
  that they are not alone with the patient.

 Make a Note

When seeking to examine any patient at any time, ensure you have
permission. It is good practice to ask if you can proceed.

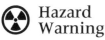 Hazard
Warning

Ensure that the practice has a strategy for managing any amorous
advances by a patient. In a group practice arrange for the patient to be
seen in future by a dentist of the opposite sex from the 'target' dentist.

The practice principal or practice owner should write to the patient
(especially if not prepared to accept the change of dentist) explaining
that attention to the dentist in question is neither appreciated nor
reciprocated.

If problem persists, warn of refusal to treat further and de-registration
from the list, explaining why and reaffirming the unwillingness of the
dentist in question to reciprocate. A private patient should be told that no
further treatment could be provided.

If a single-handed practice, the dentist should immediately write to the
patient advising that advances are not appreciated or reciprocated and
that the patient cannot continue to receive treatment at the practice. In
the case of an NHS patient the health authority should be notified
immediately. Be sure to write in confidence and describe the
circumstances as a 'professional relational difficulty'. Don't go into detail
or you may find yourself saddled with a defamation case – even if you are
right!

CHAPERONES AND AMOROUS PATIENTS

Don't argue/delay/vacillate – just sort it

- Is a chaperone available for any patient who requires one?
- Is the availability of a chaperone publicised in the waiting room or in the practice leaflet?
- Does the practice have a strategy for managing amorous patients?
- Does the practice nurse understand the significance of her role as a chaperone?
- Does the nurse ensure that the dentist is not left alone without the dentist's agreement?
- Does the dentist have any sort of signal to indicate to the nurse that he/she should not be left alone at any time with the patient?

CLINICAL PRACTICE MANAGEMENT

LET'S GET THE BASICS RIGHT

No apologies for starting with the Janet and John stuff. You'd be surprised by the number of practices that overlook the basics or forget about the renewal of some vital certificate or insurance.

Here's a check list of the basic stuff. Copy these pages and turn them into a renewal reminder.

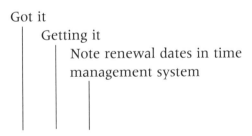

Got it

   Getting it

      Note renewal dates in time management system

- Annual practising certificates for the dentists.
- A policy for providing contractually guaranteed indemnity.
- Practising certificate for the hygienist.

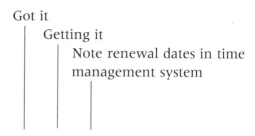

Got it
　　Getting it
　　　　Note renewal dates in time
　　　　management system

- Training certificates as appropriate
  for practice staff.
- Employer's liability insurance
  certificate (which must be
  displayed).
- Necessary practice insurance
  including public liability.
- Data protection registration.
- Arrangements for clinical waste
  collection and disposal.
- TV licence (if necessary).
- COSHH assessment.
- Radiation survey/safety log.
- Autoclave and compressor
  maintenance inspection, certificate
  and programme of maintenance.
- Health and safety poster displayed.
- First aid kit.
- Accident book.
- Contracts of employment.
- Performing rights licence for
  playing music.

Wait, you're not finished yet.

Does the practice have:

- a job description for each employee including written terms of
  employment, job location, payment arrangements, holiday and sickness
  arrangements, pension arrangements and duration of employment? It
  should also include the notice period, and arrangements for the
  grievance and disciplinary arrangements?
- a job description/associate agreement for each associate?

- a contract for each associate?
- arrangements for regular staff meetings?
- protective clothing for staff if required?
- General Dental Council continuing professional development requirements?
- arrangements to keep a record of all sickness and a mechanism for collection of certificates?

STANDARD OF CARE

Time to start *talking serious* for a moment. Make a cup of coffee, come back and read this next bit carefully. The NHS is undergoing a quality make-over. Clinical governance, continuing professional development, service frameworks, clinical protocols, pronouncements by the National Institute for Clinical Excellence and all sorts of other stuff are starting to shine bright lights into dark corners.

The standard of care expected of a general dental practitioner is what is *regarded as reasonable* and what would be *provided by the prudent practitioner* under the *same or similar circumstances*. If you've read the beginning of this book, those words will ring a bell (or they should) the Bolam decision is at the heart of it.

However, because of the ever-changing nature of dentistry and the development of new materials and techniques, the acceptable or reasonable standard of care will clearly change over time. It was, for example, not so long ago that only standard Black's cavity preparations would be acceptable. Now, other forms of restoration have made the Black's technique obsolete in some circumstances.

In the event of a claim against a dentist, then those practitioners called as experts will be required to judge what a reasonable practitioner would have done in the circumstances. The level of *skill* against which the judgement will be made, depends upon what procedure the dental practitioner was undertaking. If the procedure was one that would normally be undertaken by a general dental practitioner, the standard against which he will be measured is that of the ordinarily skilled general dental practitioner. If the procedure is one that would normally be undertaken by a consultant or specialist, then he will be judged against the standard of an ordinarily skilled specialist in that area.

 Make a Note

The specialist with which a general practitioner would be compared would be one appearing on the GDC's specialist list.

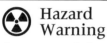 **Hazard Warning**

Any general dental practitioner has a responsibility to maintain his knowledge in those areas in which he provides treatment by undergoing suitable educational activities. Failure to maintain up-to-date knowledge and the continuation of unproven or outdated procedures with materials no longer regarded as of an adequate standard are likely to result in an allegation of poor performance to the General Dental Council. In the event of a claim for negligence, failure to demonstrate knowledge of modern techniques may count against the practitioner.

VICARIOUS LIABILITY

There's a phrase to conjure with. What does it mean?

A general dental practitioner has *vicarious liability* for his employed staff. This means the dentist is responsible for their acts and omissions and may therefore have to pay any damages arising from those acts and omissions.

Ouch! You can see it is an important concept because, even in those circumstances where the dentist maintains a perfectly good standard, an action of a member of the staff who negligently causes a patient injury, may result in the dentist being liable. The liability extends to all staff within the general dental practitioner's team.

 Make a Note

The fact that a general dental practitioner may be held to be an independent contractor is not relevant if he is the employer.

Dentists should think of an employee's professional actions as an extension of their own. Be sure that all the staff clearly understand this.

How can the dentist be sure staff act in a certain way and 'get it right first time', particularly when working unsupervised? Easy, a one word answer:

Protocols

Protocols are the railroad track of management. They are the map, the road-sign and the path to follow. Protocols should spell out, step, by step, how a task should be approached, the elements of carrying it out and the standard of outcome that is expected. For example, in the case of the reception staff, protocols should be provided, detailing what should be done in all aspects of the work, including:

- making appointments
- taking telephone messages
- accepting requests for domiciliary visits
- payment management instructions.

Similar protocols will be especially important for any supporting dental staff including associates, assistants, dental hygienists and others.

Education, education, education. Or, in the words of the medical profession, training, training and training – is the answer. Tell people what is expected of them, train them to do it, check they are doing it, all the time, every time.

All new staff should be fully trained in their roles. Failure to provide adequate training leaves the dentist very vulnerable to the possibility of a complaint or claim on the basis of his liability for staff actions.

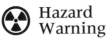 **Hazard Warning**

No task should be delegated to a member of staff unless they have been fully trained to undertake it and, if appropriate, a protocol on how to undertake the activity clearly demonstrated to them.

REDUCING THE RISKS OF VICARIOUS LIABILITY

So, you find yourself trying to unravel a complaint from a patient about the treatment they have received from one of your staff. You have no idea about the issue because it involves only staff members and the patient(s).

If your staff have clear protocols and they have been breached during the incident that led to the complaint, there may be a case for disciplinary action against the staff member for failure to comply with protocols. The important thing is this. If you know how the job should have been done, and there are clear protocols that describe what is expected, then you have some idea about what did, or didn't go wrong. Were the protocols followed, abandoned, or not in place? Staff who commit errors in patient management cannot be criticised if there are no clear instructions on how the tasks should be carried out. As the dentist's reputation can depend on the performance of the staff, getting the right people around you starts to take on a new significance.

When choosing staff, ensure that the recruitment process has some expert input. Before starting the process, ensure that:

- you know the role the appointee is expected to fulfil
- you prepare a job description that contains **every** element to be expected of the employee.

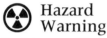 **Hazard Warning**

Problems will arise if the job that you want done does not match what the employee was expecting to do.

At the interview there are four key things to find out.

- Does the applicant understand the scope of the job?
- Can they do the job?
- Do they have the qualifications for the job?
- Is the potential employee a 'team player'?

 Make a Note

Appointments should be provisional dependent upon satisfactory references, which should always be pursued. You might find out more if you have a telephone conversation with a referee. Some folks don't like writing down what they really think! A period of mutual assessment (say three months) may be useful.

Here are five employment rules – follow these and sleep easier!

1   Think of the employee's professional actions as extensions of your own. Make sure that the staff also view their actions in this way.

2 The dentist should ensure that he sets the tone for the behaviour of his staff by ensuring adequate training and protocols. Such protocols should be in the form of a written policy manual to define the limits of staff roles and to formalise patient follow-up procedures.

3 Ensure that professional liability insurance includes vicarious liability. Be certain that the cover is guaranteed and not discretionary.

4 Ensure that, if any new dentist joins the practice as an associate or an assistant, the dentist demonstrates that he is on the professional register of the General Dental Council and that he has a suitable guaranteed indemnity for insurance.

5 When employing any new member of staff, make sure that you check on their curriculum vitae and that you follow up references etc.

STANDARDS CHECKLIST

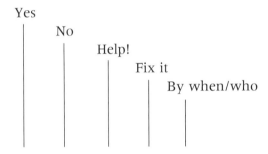

Yes

No

Help!

Fix it

By when/who

• Does the dentist maintain skills and knowledge in the areas in which he provides treatment?

• Does the dentist understand that he is liable for the acts and omissions of his employed staff?

• Does the dentist have clear protocols for staff including making appointments, taking telephone messages, accepting patients for domiciliary visits and managing patient payments?

• Does the dentist provide comprehensive staff training?

MANAGING PATIENT EXPECTATIONS

Great expectations – a Dickens of an idea.

In this 24-hour, seven days a week, I want it now, gimme everything society – what of the poor old dentist trying to drill out a living? The whole of the NHS is under pressure from a consumerised society and the question is, can a public service meet expectations in a market driven world?

Patients often have high expectations about what they think the dentist should achieve for them. This is particularly true when they have cosmetic dental defects or when they have facial characteristics that they attribute to a dental cause.

However, the expectations don't stop there! They may include the availability of parking, the comfort and privacy of the waiting area, the expectation of confidentiality when dealing with a receptionist and the level of courtesy and friendliness that they expect to be afforded to them by other members of the practice staff.

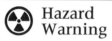 **Hazard Warning**

Complaints and claims often arise because the dentist does not meet the patient's expectations. It is important in any first consultation to be sure that the patient clearly explains to you what they do expect and, if it is not possible to meet those expectations, that's the time to say so!

Misleading articles in magazines or word of mouth advice may have led the patient to a belief that a particular form of treatment is either available or likely to be successful, when it is not. Dentists should not assume that patients understand anything about dentistry. It is frequently the case that even simple procedures are not understood or misunderstood by a patient seeking dental treatment.

During the process of providing a protracted course of treatment, it is important to regularly review the patient's expectations. The difference between what the dentist can deliver and what the patient can expect may be described as the 'negligence gap'.

Here are a few phrases that sound like a compensation claim in the making:

- 'We can give you a film star smile'
- 'We can cater for even the most cowardly patient'
- 'We guarantee that you will not feel a thing'.

Make a Note

If, at the outset, it becomes apparent that you and the patient are not going to get along because the patient has expectations that you can't deliver, tell the patient and let them go with no charge.

Here are some common problems from the *'expectation zone'*:

• Mixing of treatment. The requirement for sorts of treatment which are not within the scope of the National Health Service although the patient does not wish to receive treatment privately.
• Treatments where the patient asks for sedation or anaesthetic that is not available in the practice.
• Treatment of a nature or complexity that requires care beyond the dentist.
• The request for treatment in such a way or in a particular sequence that the dentist does not feel is either clinically acceptable or reasonable.
• Patient requests for appointments at times when the dentist is not available, e.g. Saturday afternoons.
• Circumstances where the patient appears rude, aggressive or generally unpleasant or is simply someone that the dentist really does not feel he wants to treat.

 Hazard Warning

It is very important not to discriminate against any patient on grounds of ethnicity, religion or sexual orientation. Dentists should not refuse to treat those patients who are HIV positive.

Get things straight right from the start – so everyone knows where they are.

When making an appointment to see a patient, it is important to make clear any practice policies that will impinge upon that patient's treatment. These include:

• arrangements for payment
• arrangements for making and cancelling appointments
• information if appropriate on the necessary duration of appointments
• expectations when appropriate about what will be accomplished at each appointment.

Whatever it is, *'tell it early and tell it often'*. Perception is everything. How you see it may not be how the patient sees it.

Look at it this way . . .

Dentist	Patient
Reasonable clinical standards	Does it match expectations?
Reasonable outcome	How long will it take?
Prompt and complete payment	How much will it cost?
Effective anaesthesia	Will it hurt?
Notification to the patient of any standards which cannot be met.	Will I look good to those people who see me?

Matching what the dentist can deliver against what the patient hopes for is the trick to ensure a minimum risk of disappointment, failure, refusal to pay and possible litigation.

 Make a Note

Think of the patient as a customer – then think about how you like to be treated and motivate the whole team to develop and maintain a customer focus.

The patient as a customer? How do you feel about that? Does the surgery present like a Marks and Sparks shop? Does the practice look presentable and welcoming.

Are . . .

- the premises well maintained?
- waiting room seats adequate?
- privacy and confidentiality maintained?
- toilet facilities adequate and of good quality?
- consulting rooms efficient and comfortable looking?
- there facilities to notify patients of delays in appointments?

Also check this out:

Have you got the usual pile of brochures in reception – are they up to date, well presented and do they include information about:

Yup

- the practice
- the practice telephone numbers
- the dentists and the staff
- the general dental services that are provided
- any specialist services that are provided, e.g. cosmetic work or implants
- opening hours of the practice
- public transport and parking arrangements
- the provision of care in an emergency
- arrangements for NHS patients and patients who are being treated privately
- any treatment exclusions
- the policy if an appointment is missed or cancelled without adequate warning.

 Make a Note

Private patients? Identify whether the patient has insurance, e.g. Denplan, and give the patient any help-line number.

Services any good?

Of course they are! Really? How do you know?

How about asking the customers (sorry, patients). Try a patient questionnaire. Be sure it includes these top line issues.

- Review of services provided.
- The opportunity for patients to record services not provided.
- Costs of treatment.
- Attitude of dentist and staff.
- Ways practice can be improved.

MANAGING PATIENT EXPECTATIONS . . .

And avoiding the risks associated with disappointment.

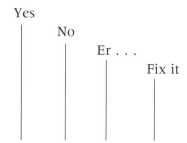

Yes

No

Er . . .

Fix it

- Does the dentist recognise the problems
  associated with meeting patient expectations?
- Does the dentist avoid making inflated or
  unattainable claims for his or her work?
- Does the dentist have a policy for managing
  patients whose expectations cannot be met? Is
  it documented?
- Does the dentist have a clear policy to avoid
  any sort of discrimination?
- Does the dentist provide patient questionnaires
  to review his patient activity?

And the staff? Frontline staff are the shop window of the practice. Don't
overlook how hard it is to be permanently pleasant! Especially at the end of
a long day or if there's trouble at home.

Encourage staff to have a customer focus and to bring to work the
expectations they have in the world outside the practice. Don't forget
their training needs.

Is the receptionist:

- courteous and with a friendly manner?
- able to act as patient friend, adviser and supporter?
- able to act as an ambassador for the practice?
- able to negotiate and have management skills?
- good on the telephone?
- dressed in a professional manner, clean and smart?

All too obvious and basic? You must be joking! The problem is no
receptionist is daft enough to be rude, or off-hand with the dentist.

Therefore, dentists imagine receptionists are equally lovely to the patients. Try a test. Take 10p out of the practice petty cash, go down the road and ring yourself up! Stand-by for a surprise!

 Make a Note

Are receptionists clear how to deal with a complaining patient quickly? Can they avoid disturbance and upset to other patients who may be present? Dealing with difficult people is an art. Arrange some training . . .

 Hazard Warning

Are you clear about the demarcation between private and NHS treatments. To mix treatments is dangerous unless you have a full understanding of the terms of service and the NHS regulations. Using excuses not to provide some NHS treatments on the grounds of cost is both fraudulent and unethical.

Done some work and can't get paid?

Do you have a policy for managing bad debts? Issues will include:

- Is the sum outstanding actually worth collecting?
- If it is a substantial sum, will the patient counterclaim (with justification are you prepared for a fight)?

Each case should be managed on its merits and the blanket referral of any bad debts to a debt-collection agency may not always be the best idea. Try a personal approach, try negotiation and don't forget the small claims court. Cheap and easy to do.

 Make a Note

If you do use a debt collecting agency check out if they have experience in dealing with patients, can they tell you about other practices they have collected debts for – check 'em out!

And don't forget, make it easy to pay and you'll probably get paid.

- Are there suitable facilities for making payments?
- Does the receptionist have access to clear information in order to ensure that the patient is charged the correct amount?

- Is there a private area within the reception where the patient and the receptionist can discuss money without other patients overhearing the discussion?
- Does the practice accept credit cards and is there a mechanism for verifying the validity of a card?
- Is there an area away from reception where a patient can be taken if a dispute arises about payment or the patient feels that a payment is inappropriate in respect of a particular item of treatment?

EMERGENCY SERVICES

No dentist should be allowed to become a dentist until they've had crippling toothache at 3 am on a Sunday!

Well, perhaps not. But emergency services are an out-of-hours problem for dentists and a real pain for the customers or patients, if you prefer!

Getting emergency services right:

During normal hours:

- an arrangement for a patient to be seen promptly if an emergency arises
- an emergency number on an answering machine if the practice is closed at lunchtime.

Out-of-hours:

- an emergency number where the patient can seek help at any time in an emergency
- the dentist should be contactable without the patient having to ring more than two numbers
- if the dentist is unavailable, a deputy should be available to provide cover.

In the event of a medical emergency in the surgery, the dentist should ensure that:

- all staff are fully trained to deal with any emergency that may arise
- life support equipment is available and everyone understands how it is used and whose role involves the use of particular items of equipment or drugs.

Training should be regularly refreshed and revisited.

- ensure that the management of emergencies is carried out professionally and efficiently, promptly and without any panic
- ensure that every member of staff understands what their own role will be
- ensure that staff are skilled in the management of common medical conditions and the use of any equipment which is available.

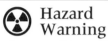 **Hazard Warning**

The conditions for which training should be given should include faints, angina, diabetic pre-coma and coma, epilepsy, myocardial infarct, stroke, acute allergy and the inhalation of foreign bodies.

The value of a good general medical questionnaire to be completed by every patient joining the practice and updated with every new course is considerable.

Cut this out and use it as a checklist for your emergency kit.

The Emergency Kit

The kit should contain:
- A portable oxygen cylinder
- A Brook Airway (contains a one-way valve – more pleasant than mouth-to-mouth resuscitation) or the new universal airway, the Combitube
- Ventilation Bag (Ambubag)
- Defibrillator (at present only if GA used but becoming more common and dentist should consider if happy to do so. If available the staff must be trained in its use)
- Disposable 2ml and 5ml syringes
- Disposable pink and green needles
- Injections of:
    - Adrenaline 1:1000 (1mg/ml)
    - Diazepam 10mg/2ml
    - Glucose 50ml
    - Glucagon 1mg
    - Hydrocortisone 100mg (with sterile water for injection)
- Tablets:
    - Antihistamine
    - Soluble Aspirin
- Glyceryl Trinitrate Spray
- Salbutamol Inhaler

It is vital that the nature and use of all drugs in the kit is fully understood.

⚠️ Hazard
Warning

The kit must be inspected regularly and any expiry dates checked. The date of checking should be recorded on the kit. The kit should be easily accessible to any staff member at any time. All staff should be trained in contacting the ambulance service if an ambulance is required. The procedure to be adopted should be recorded on a card placed at every telephone point.

EMERGENCY TELEPHONE PROCEDURE

Dial 999. Ask for ambulance service. Be ready to give:

• your name and name of practice
• address of practice
• telephone number of practice

'We require an ambulance urgently.'

Give brief details of the patient's symptoms and signs, e.g. collapse, breathlessness, chest pain, agitation, fits, loss of consciousness, vomiting.

Answer any further questions which the ambulance control may ask clearly and concisely. Do not panic.

If the practice is difficult to find, provide directions,
e.g. 'Coming from the ambulance station it is the third turning on the left after the supermarket.'

Note the time of the call request.

It may be a wise precaution to leave the details of the route to the practice and a suitable map at the local Ambulance station.

TRAINING FOR THE UNEXPECTED?

Here are the most common incidents that the dentist and appropriate staff should be trained and practised in dealing with:

• Angina
• Myocardial infarction

- Cardiac Arrest
- Cerebro-vascular accident
- Fainting
- Epileptic fit
- Collapse of unknown origin
- Diabetic hypoglycaemic coma
- Allergic reactions
- Anaphylactic shock
- Inhalation of a foreign body.

Training should include cardio-pulmonary resuscitation. All staff should be able to place a patient in the recovery position.

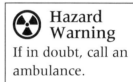

Hazard Warning
If in doubt, call an ambulance.

The minimum number of staff required to cope with an emergency must be clearly understood. In some circumstances two may be insufficient and the training must reflect the circumstances.

EMERGENCY SERVICES CHECKLIST

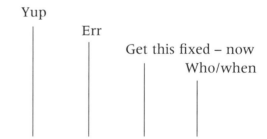

Yup

Err

Get this fixed – now

Who/when

- Does the practice ensure that all dentists and staff have regular training in the management of medical emergencies?
- Does the practice have life support equipment available? Does anyone know how to use it?
- Does the practice staff know how to perform cardio-pulmonary resuscitation?

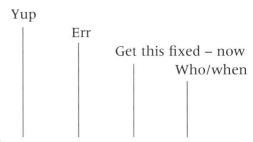

Yup

Err

Get this fixed – now

Who/when

- Is the dentist familiar with the use of all the drugs in the emergency kit? Are all drug expiry dates checked regularly?
- Is the emergency kit easily accessible?
- Does the practice have emergency oxygen and are the cylinders checked regularly and refilled as necessary?
- Are the rubber components of masks, *Ambubags*, etc. regularly checked in case of perishing?
- Does the emergency kit contain all relevant telephone numbers in case assistance is required?
- Does the dentist have an emergency telephone procedure known to all staff and able to be used by any staff member contacting the emergency services?
- Is the procedure in the form of a notice and kept by the telephone?

DENTAL TREATMENT

DENTAL TREATMENT

Well, it's what you want to do, isn't it? But it's a risky business. Here are a few things to plant the seeds of insomnia!

1   Infection control (that's dealt with in the section on health and safety).
2   Sterilisation procedures (that's in the health and safety section, too).
3   Dental equipment.

Common sense tells you that the standard of equipment within the surgery is of crucial importance and not just for safety reasons. It's expensive and represents a sizeable capital investment. It's in everyone's interest to look after it.

Programmes of regular maintenance should be prepared and maintained at all times. All instruments should be inspected regularly to ensure that they are free from defects.

If an instrument breaks or there is some form of failure that results in injury to the patient, the instrument, including the broken part or fragment, should be carefully retained for future inspection. If it were shown that the equipment was intrinsically defective, then any claim arising out

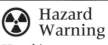 **Hazard Warning**

Hand instruments that demonstrate any form of corrosion should be discarded.

Hand pieces, where the friction retention of burs becomes in any way loose, should be withdrawn from use and repaired or discarded.

of a patient injury would then be directed at the instrument manufacturer rather than at the dentist. Phew . . .

Special attention should be provided to X-ray units, compressors and sterilisation facilities. X-ray equipment must comply with health and safety requirements (there's more about this on page 179). No matter how minor the defects in the machine or in the developing facilities, remember, they could result in a production of poor images that may in turn result in failed diagnoses and consequent errors in treatment.

Got a compressor? Check it out . . .

A compressor failure without adequate back up or through insufficient maintenance may have serious consequences if it occurs in the middle of a complex or prolonged treatment. Failure to be able to maintain aspiration or to complete preparation of a tooth or teeth may cause considerable difficulty. It may not be possible to

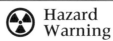 **Hazard Warning**

Sterilisation is vitally important, particularly in an era where Hepatitis B and HIV infection have attained such importance.

provide temporary restorations that are adequate and there may be a risk that the patient will be left in pain. Accumulation of saliva may have serious consequences if the patient suffers acute discomfort.

Ensure adequate sterilisation.

* Instruments should be carefully scrubbed, followed by autoclaving.
* Have colour sensitive recording facilities to ensure that the autoclave effectively completes its cycle when instruments are being sterilised.
* Retain the indicator tapes – essential in defending a dentist where it is alleged that a patient contracted a particular infection during dental treatment at the practice.

No matter what they say, there is no satisfactory substitute for an autoclave.

 Make a Note

Retain all monitoring, servicing and repairs information as evidence of good care and maintenance.

PRIVACY

No one looks their best lying almost horizontal with a mouthful of dental instruments! Keeping the surgery door closed when appropriate is obvious.

Not so obvious is ensuring that conversations within the surgery cannot be heard outside, even when the door is closed.

What about conversations between staff members? The patient should not be able to hear conversations between staff members about matters relating to that patient or any other patient, their medical history, decisions about the dental treatment provided or the payment arrangements. Make sure you cannot be overheard.

THE LABORATORY AND HYGIENE ARRANGEMENTS

Patient infections might be passed on to technicians because of micro-organisms that may have been left on a prosthesis following contact with patient's saliva. That can lead to all laboratory instruments, machinery and services that come into contact with the prosthesis becoming infected. Equally, any infection acquired in the laboratory may be transmitted back to the patient when the prosthesis is fitted. Nasty!

So, ensure there is:

- a process for disinfecting all restorations, prostheses and appliances before they are touched by the laboratory technician or returned to the patient
- an effective hygiene protocol within the laboratory to ensure that there is no risk of cross-contamination of patients.

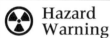 **Hazard Warning**

Patients may be sensitive to some of the chemicals and other materials used in the laboratory. It is therefore important that all ultrasonic cleaning fluids, detergents and disinfectants, pumice and rouges should be thoroughly removed from all appliances before being returned to the patient.

EXAMINATION AND DIAGNOSIS

PATIENT DENTAL RECORDS

Good quality records are good for you! They:

- help you to provide high quality dentistry
- give you a solid defence to any complaint or claim.

Remember the rules. Records must be:

* accurate
* complete
* legible.

Don't overlook the fact that notes may be used by any members of the dental team. Good notes provide a vital source of information. However good you think your memory is, it isn't as good as a set of notes!

Here's what should be in a set of patient notes:

Patient Personal Information – all the obvious stuff . . .

 Make a Note

Abbreviations, particularly obscure abbreviations, should be avoided and there should be no disparaging comments of any sort included in the notes.

* name
* address
* telephone contacts
* family information if appropriate
* marital status.

 Make a Note

Ensure that information about the family of minors, including details of custody in foster cases or information where divorce has occurred is fully recorded.

Let's make some history.

HEALTH HISTORY

The notes should contain a comprehensive medical history. The dentist will normally note this on the first visit.

Be sure to include any relevant medical conditions:

* heart disease
* hypertension

- diabetes
- drug therapy
- systemic diseases with oral manifestations.

Ask the patient whether there is any medical reason why they have been advised not to have particular sorts of dental treatment or whether any precautions have been advised before starting.

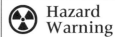 **Hazard Warning**

If you have any doubts at all about the physical health of the patient – stop and seek permission to contact the patient's general practitioner for further information.

It is important that the medical history is reliable. Get it wrong and you end up with significant patient injury.

Every time a patient attends, the dentist should always ask the three 'keep you out of trouble' questions:

1   Have you seen a doctor or other healthcare professional since your last consultation?
2   Have you suffered any illness or injury?
3   Have you stopped, started or changed any medication?

DENTAL HISTORY

Ever wondered why a patient has chosen your practice? Is it your stunning good looks, your sartorial elegance, your winning smile or your engaging conversation? Could it be because you are a good dentist? Could it be you're local, accessible or come highly recommended?

Try to understand the events that may have lead to the patient joining the practice. Ask a sensitive question or two. Is there dissatisfaction with the previous dentist? What makes him or her think you can do any better? Is there an on-going problem that the patient believes you can sort out?

Think about asking:

- why the patient has changed dentist
- what the patient has been told about current dental state and any existing diagnoses
- the dates of treatment and provision of current restorations and appliances
- whether the patient was treated as an NHS patient or privately.

Ask the right question and you'll find out about the patient's expectations. Are there any irreconcilable differences between the patient's expectations and your ability to deliver?

Is it worth trying to be a hero? If it looks like a difficult patient who's swapped from dentist to dentist, or looks like grief, do you really want to be the next dentist on the list? Be brave enough to say *no, thanks*.

SOCIAL HISTORY

All very holistic! But it is important to get to grips with and is information that might impact on providing therapy, costs or time constraints.
  Let's get to it!

THE EXAMINATION

The first examination is the foundation for all subsequent examinations. Must get this one especially right. Look for:

• teeth present and teeth missing
• existing dental restorations
• appliances and their condition
• the periodontal status. *It is important to record a base line periodontal pocket charting at the first visit.*
• occlusion
• any temporo-mandibular joint disorders
• any dental caries or other pathology of the teeth and soft tissues
• any known previous X-ray results.

 Make a Note

Where you can, it is important to make positive statements. The omission of a note on the basis that the situation is 'normal' may result in difficulty proving that a particular examination was actually done subsequently. Do it all and make a note of it all.

DENTAL MODELS

Dental models are often very valuable in demonstrating pre-treatment dental disorders and may enable the dentist to demonstrate both how cosmetic improvements may be achieved and how functional anomalies can be corrected. Treat models like dental records and keep them for the same time. Running out of space? Well, maybe you can keep them for a bit of a shorter period. But, if you can, hang onto them.

ASSESSING THE QUALITY OF ANOTHER DENTIST'S TREATMENT

Tricky this. No one likes to be critical of another professional. Perhaps a patient will ask, informally, what you think about the treatment that has been pro-

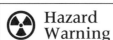 **Hazard Warning**

It is frequently the case that complaints or claims arise from failure to diagnose dental disease, periodontal disease, oral cancer and other dental conditions. The dentist will often remember discussions with the patient but the dental record does not support this. So engrave this onto your brain-box 'IF IT WASN'T DOCUMENTED IT WASN'T DONE'. If the information is not on the dental record then you have two chances defending your actions – slim and none!

vided previously. The dentist's primary obligation is to explain current treatment needs by assessing current oral health status. The dentist should recommend the required current treatment. There is no requirement for a dentist to judge any suggestion of negligence or a previous dentist.

Avoid getting drawn into a tricky situation. Don't guess at why a dentist undertook a particular course of treatment. If a patient enquires why a particular item of treatment needs to be re-done or why a previous dentist failed to recognise an oral condition, make it clear that you were not present at the time and were not examining the signs which then existed. Explain that you're not in a position to make a comment on why the previous dentist took a particular action.

If you need to know about previous treatment then write or telephone. It is important not to make 'off the cuff' comments about a dental state with an implication that a previous dentist may have been in some way responsible. Patients listen very carefully and it may be that casual or unguarded remarks may result in the launch of a complaint against a previous practitioner. In those circumstances it could be what you said that kicked the whole thing off. And, you're likely to become entangled in any subsequent actions.

It is important to remember that, where there is insufficient information to make a definite assessment, the dentist is under no obligation to guess the reason why completed dental treatment appears as it does, no matter how much the patient insists on obtaining that information.

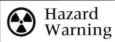 **Hazard Warning**

Don't think all this means you have to be dishonest with a patient to protect a colleague. You have a responsibility to the patient and to the General Dental Council not to conceal questionable or poor quality dental care. However, this doesn't mean jumping to conclusions about the circumstances under which particular items of treatment were provided or about the dentist who provided it. Providing dentistry of an appropriate standard protects the patient. Keeping thorough dental records both about your treatment and that provided by a previous dentist protects you.

THE DENTAL HYGIENIST

Hygienists have now become a permanent and expected part of the services offered by most practices. Hygienists can provide a valuable second opinion and, by the nature of their costs and training, are able to provide a more comprehensive service than the dentist in many circumstances. However, remember that the responsibility for the patient remains with you, the dentist. You are liable for any acts or omissions of a hygienist you employ.

The circumstances may be different for self-employed hygienists who have their own indemnity cover.

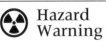 **Hazard Warning**

Don't abrogate responsibility to the hygienist. Make sure that you examine the periodontium when seeing the patient for other dental care. Ensure that NHS claims and private charging are correctly based.

EXAMINATION AND DIAGNOSIS CHECKLIST

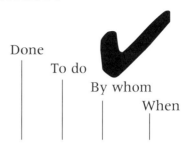

Done
    To do
        By whom
           When

- Ensure that dental records are accurate, complete and legible.
- Are abbreviations avoided?
- Ensure that no pejorative, racist or other inappropriate comments are recorded in the notes.
- Do records routinely include all necessary personal information?
- Do records include medical history noted at the first visit?
- At each new attendance is the medical history up-dated?
- Do you take a full dental history including details of other dentists who have provided treatment?
- Do you undertake a full examination including a full periodontal assessment?
- Do you remain alert to patient dissatisfaction with the work of a previous dentist?
- Do you refrain from making any comments about a previous dentist's work?
- Do you understand that he or she retains responsibility for the work delegated to the hygienist?

RADIOLOGY

Radiography is a routine part of dental practice – how did you ever manage without it? However, don't take the kit for granted. Why?
Because:

- many diagnoses depend on the acquisition of high quality radiographs for their confirmation
- the investigations are associated with the use of ionising radiations and they are not without hazard either to patient or operator.

Radiographic and radiological techniques should operate according to a series of protocols and guidelines. This means that rigid policies relating to the use and maintenance of radiological equipment and good practice must be used when undertaking radiographic examinations.

IONISING RADIATIONS

No radiographic exposure is without health hazards although for most dental investigations this is very small. Nevertheless, radiographic exposures must be kept as small as possible.

The voltage, the method by which the ionising radiation is generated, the methods by which it is filtered and collimated and the type of film and its sensitivity also has an impact on the quantity of radiation.

The machine should be regularly inspected to ensure that it complies with all health and safety requirements. Dump high dosage machines as soon as possible and treat yourself to some modern kit.

Guess how many radiographic examinations general dental practitioners undertake every year? Ten million, 15 million or 20 million?

Answer: about 20

To put the doses and hazards in context, the amount of radiation supplied with X-rays should be compared with the ordinary background radiation to which we are all constantly exposed.

Think of it this way:

- A chest X-ray is equal to about three to four days of background radiation.

- A panoral X-ray is equivalent to about four to five days of background radiation.
- Bitewings are equivalent to about one day of background radiation.

PANORAL RADIOGRAPHY

Panoral radiographs use more ionising radiation than other dental techniques. It is therefore important that the X-ray is correctly positioned and of the highest quality. Take care in positioning and processing the radiograph. Poor quality or defective radiographs lead to reduction in the value of the examination in making diagnostic and prognostic decisions.

In orthodontics, a panoral X-ray may provide comprehensive information about the existing and developing dentition. However, it should not be regarded as a routine procedure in all patients but only where extensive orthodontic treatment dictates that a general examination is required.

For oral surgery, a panoral X-ray may provide valuable information in terms of the inclination and the degree of

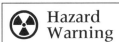 **Hazard Warning**

A panoral radiograph should not be regarded as appropriate for every new patient even if the dentition is heavily restored. Such an X-ray should be taken only if there is a specific indication. If the patient is edentulous, the only indication for routine panoral screen is when clinical examination suggests bony pathology or where implant surgery is contemplated.

rotation of lower third molars and will also indicate the extent of various types of periapical and other bony lesions. In many incidences, particularly in respect of the extraction of fully erupted teeth, periapical X-rays are of higher quality and more reliable than panoral.

So now you know! And, by the way . . .

In temporo-mandibular joint dysfunction, it is very rare for radiography to reveal any pathology. Such investigations should be confined to investigation within secondary care where there is a history of trauma or in anticipation of the need for some sort of corrective surgery.

CHILDREN'S RADIOLOGY

Got kids? Know any? Well, you must have been one! They're different! They wriggle about, cry, are easily frightened and might bite your finger! They can also be fun and very rewarding to treat.

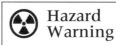 **Hazard Warning**

Children provide specific, and often quite difficult, diagnostic problems, particularly in respect of the developing dentition. The issues may revolve around the presence or absence of particular teeth and for orthodontic planning purposes.

It is of course vital that the radiation dosage should be kept as low as possible for all children at all times. In many cases, a small number of simple X-rays will suffice. Radiographic examination will seldom be required in general practice for any child below the age of 7.

There are however, a number of indications for taking X-rays where a clinical examination or past history leaves suspicion that there may be an abnormality that will impair or disrupt the occlusion or the development of the oral facial skeleton.

Such factors include:

- a history of hypodontia
- a history of trauma
- an unusual eruption pattern
- delayed appearance of teeth or unexplained missing teeth
- clinically impacted teeth
- unusual tooth morphology
- unexplained hard dentoalveolar swelling
- mobility of teeth
- facial asymmetry
- traumatic occlusion
- first molars, poor long term prognosis.

In the continued management of children or if referral is required, new radiographs should only be taken if previous radiographic information is no longer sufficient to provide the necessary information for clinical management.

> 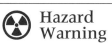 **Hazard**
> **Warning**
>
> In ongoing orthodontic treatment, there may be a need to take radiographs as the treatment proceeds in order to ensure that the dental and supporting tissues are healthy and that a tooth or teeth are erupting in a satisfactory manner.
>
> If orthodontics is being managed using fixed appliances, then regular X-rays may be required as the only effective way of monitoring progress adequately. The radiographs selected should reflect the fact that there is risk of root resorption associated with movement of teeth.
>
> At the end of treatment and during retention periods, there may be a necessity to offer further radiography. However, each case should be carefully assessed and the X-ray should only be taken if there is a clear indication for doing so.

DENTAL CARIES

Spare a thought for the days of dentistry when there was no radiology!

Today, radiography is essential in the diagnosis of dental caries particularly when size of lesion or location preclude its discovery by clinical examination. Periodic bitewing examinations can also contribute to care planning or preventive and operative dental care. The number of bitewing examinations must be sufficient to avoid the risk that lesions will be missed. The frequency of such radiographic examinations will depend on:

- age
- caries experience
- the rate of development of caries
- lesions of the individual.

It is reasonable to take bitewing X-rays at an initial examination for all children identified of being of high caries risk. Continuing six monthly examinations in that group should also be carried out, although the rate of caries incidence should be monitored so that a reduction is accompanied by a reduced frequency of radiography. Reduced frequency of

> 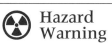 **Hazard**
> **Warning**
>
> Such radiographs should never be taken as a way of pre-empting or avoiding any sort of clinical examination. They should be regarded only as an adjunct to the process. Routine radiographs taken simply because time has elapsed since the last X-rays is not supportable.

radiography is appropriate for those children with moderate and low caries risk.

 Make a Note

For adults, the same criteria for bitewings should be employed as for children in respect of the frequency and investigations.

FIBREOPTIC TRANSILLUMINATION

Many authorities suggest that fibreoptic transillumination can either supplement or replace bitewing radiographs.

Undoubtedly, the technique is valuable in identifying some lesions at approximal surfaces. However, bitewing X-rays will identify more dentinal and enamel lesions than FOTI only and should therefore not be used as a replacement for radiography.

PERIODONTAL ASSESSMENT

Look out! The number of complaints about failure to diagnose or the late diagnosis of periodontal conditions is on the up-and-up. It is essential to make an initial detailed periodontal assessment with every new patient and to regularly monitor any changes that may occur in the periodontal status.

And, clinical examination and radiological assessment may be helpful in the following areas.

- The conditions and levels of alveolar bone.
- The presence of pocketing.
- The presence of associated periapical disease.

 Make a Note

Bitewing X-rays may give an indication of the state of the periodontal condition but specific suspect areas should be assessed using periapical X-rays and, if the hard tissue deterioration is considered to be generalised, a panoral film may be valuable.

Ask the experts? The Faculty of General Dental Practitioners' Expert Panel make the following recommendations:

- If a patient has uniform pocketing of less than 5 mm and little or no recession, horizontal bitewings can be taken.
- If a patient is pocketing in excess of 5 mm, vertical bitewing radiographs are recommended supplemented by intraoral periapical views.
- If the patient has irregular pocketing, bitewing radiographs, horizontal or vertical depending upon pocket depth (supported by periapical radiographs), are best.
- A panoral radiograph may offer a dose advantage over large numbers of intraoral radiographs and may be considered as an alternative if available. It may be particularly so where there are concurrent problems for which radiography is necessary, i.e. symptomatic third molars, multiple existing restorations, heavily restored teeth, multiple endodontically treated teeth for patients new to the practice.

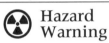 **Hazard Warning**

In periodontal disease, radiology should not be viewed as a substitute for thorough clinical examination. In heavily restored dentitions, if the tooth is to be prepared for a crown or to act as a retainer for a bridge, a periapical radiograph should be taken.

Similarly, a periapical view should be taken of any vital tooth which is to be crowned or used as a bridge abutment. Regular bitewing radiographs should be taken in those cases with high caries experience and more intermittent films used in patients with moderate or low experience. If the tooth has been root filled and is symptom free, five yearly assessments by radiography should suffice.

ENDODONTICS

Radiography is essential in endodontic therapy. When taking an X-ray before, during or at the conclusion of endodontic therapy, it is important to ensure that the picture obtained is of the highest quality because it is required not only for assessment but also for comparison with other films.

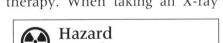 **Hazard Warning**

Endodontics should not be undertaken without access to radiographic examination.

It is therefore essential that the apex of tooth is clearly shown and that the root is not lengthened or shortened by inappropriate positioning of the film or the cone.

You must ensure:

• that the film is correctly positioned, exposed, processed and stored
• that beam alignment devices are employed
• that the films are viewed using a high quality clear light source
• that magnification is employed when viewing films.

During consideration of a tooth for endodontic therapy, and following a detailed clinical examination of the tooth including assessment of vitality, a quality periapical radiograph will provide valuable additional information in terms of the condition of the pulp, the configuration of the root(s), the presence of periapical disease and the presence of any associated periodontal conditions which might make root canal therapy less appropriate or desirable. The judgement about the value of root canal therapy can only be made by a combination of clinical and radiological examination. Clearly, the prognosis of the endodontically treated tooth must be reasonably good for such treatment to be considered.

 Make a Note

If the X-ray does not include the apex of the tooth, it is of very limited value in making any sort of assessment.

Unfavourable factors will include:

• severe periodontal bone loss
• internal or external resorption
• unfavourable root morphology, root fractures or other pathology.

Also, you need to think about:

• patient compliance and cost
• number of tooth roots
• the approximate length of the roots
• any root curvature
• any root angulation
• any sclerosis in the root canals
• the proximity or relation of any other anatomical structures
  (e.g. antrum, mandibular nerve canal)

- evidence of any previous endodontic therapy
- the whole of the periapical area.

SURGICAL ROOT CANAL TREATMENT

When surgery is required, periapical X-rays must be considered to elucidate the possibility of:

- the root link (concerning periodontal support)
- the proximity of other structures
- evidence of root fracture
- the presence of perforation
- evidence of lateral canals
- the presence of extruded root canal filling material.

 Make a Note

A radiograph which is necessary for surgery should show a wide margin of periapical tissues.

CANAL INSTRUMENTATION

It will be necessary to undertake X-rays to assess root canal length against a suitable instrument. A further radiograph should be taken immediately following insertion of the root canal filling. If more than one canal is present, it may be necessary to take more than one X-ray to obtain satisfactory views. The X-ray will provide evidence of satisfactory completion and will also provide a baseline for the assessment of the root canal treatment in the future.

RADIOLOGY CHECKLIST

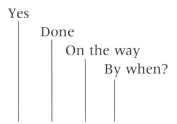

Yes
| Done
| | On the way
| | | By when?

- Is the dentist aware of all health and safety issues relating to radiology?
- Does the dentist complete a thorough history and examination of all dental and tooth bearing areas?
- Does the dentist only take radiographs in patients where action will result from radiographic findings?
- Does the dentist seek previous radiographs taken elsewhere if relevant and possible?
- Does the dentist reassess caries risk status regularly in all patients?
- Does the dentist use the appropriate radiograph treatment planning?
- Does the dentist ensure regular servicing and maintenance of any radiological equipment so that it complies with all health and safety standards?
- Does the dentist use the appropriate film in order to ensure that minimum ionising radiation is used?
- Does the dentist have adequate facilities to develop high quality radiographs?
- Does the dentist report radiographic findings in the patient notes?
- Does the dentist ensure that processing conditions are satisfactory before processing a film?
- Does the dentist ensure quality assurance in processing?

Yes
　　│ Done
　　│　│ On the way
　　│　│　│ By when?

- Does the dentist use a good quality light box for viewing together with magnifier masking out any extraneous light?
- Does the dentist mount, date, label and store all radiographs appropriately?
- Does the dentist avoid carrying out any screening or routine radiographs?
- Does the dentist avoid taking a new radiograph without examining existing films?
- Does the dentist avoid using a single or inflexible protocol for all patients?
- Does the dentist avoid using inappropriate light sources for viewing?
- Does the dentist ensure that a periapical X-ray extends at least 3 mm beyond the apex of the tooth?
- Does the dentist ensure that X-rays for surgical purposes show the condition of the tooth, root morphology, relationship of other teeth and associated structures?

TREATMENT PLANNING

Nobody plans to fail – they simply fail to plan . . .

A significant amount of dental treatment required? Better get organised and make a plan. No, not how to spend the fees received – a treatment plan! This has the advantage of laying out clearly to the patient what

 Make a Note

The treatment plan can be taken away by the patient and may be signed as a record that the patient agrees to the treatment proposed and to meet any costs associated with it.

they can expect. It is a good idea, so that the patient knows what is going to happen to them and it is a good idea for you – to get you organised. And, the plan will ensure that there is little scope for any dispute subsequently.

When planning a treatment plan here's what you should plan to have in the plan – if you see the plan?

1   Get a logical sequence. For example, if it is appropriate to provide periodontal treatment and then review in respect of providing bridge work, do not make the treatment plan in a different sequence. Especially if you are put under pressure by the patient to do work in a certain order. Stick to your plan.

2   Present all the options for treatment, even those that might differ from the dentist's preferred option or with which you may not expect the patient to agree. Do not choose a cost-based option because you feel it is the one which the patient would be able to afford.

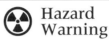 **Hazard Warning**

The treatment plan should be optimal for the patient's needs. If the patient finds the suggestion unacceptable, it is reasonable to present alternative treatment options.

However, it is unacceptable to present a treatment plan which does not secure reasonable dental health.

 Make a Note

It is up to the patient to decide whether to proceed with the treatment plan. The dentist's responsibility is to examine, diagnose and inform about treatment options.

The more lengthy or complex the treatment, the greater the need for a written treatment plan. The advantages of a treatment plan are that it will help you:

- in organising and setting priorities for treatment
- in estimating costs and time
- explain to the patient what treatment is required
- book suitable appointments
- make an estimate of the total cost
- provide evidence in the event of subsequent dispute.

Sorry to be gloomy about this but a good treatment plan can save a dentist's bacon!

TREATMENT PLANNING CHECKLIST

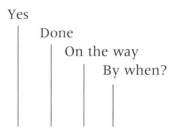

Yes
   Done
      On the way
         By when?

- Does the dentist provide a treatment plan (TP) for every patient?
- Where there is extensive treatment does the TP show the treatment in a logical sequence?
- Does the TP provide alternative options where appropriate?
- Does the plan indicate the approximate cost of each option?
- Does the dentist recognise that the patient is free to choose whichever option he or she prefers?
- Does the dentist appreciate the value of the TP in patient education, agreement to treatment and avoidance of disputes?

COSMETIC DENTISTRY

Here's the golden rule:

. . . it is unwise to disturb the dentition of a patient who is dentally fit unless there are very clear indications that the appearance *of the teeth* is giving cause for concern.

> ☢ Hazard
> ☢ Warning
>
> Very great caution must be exercised whenever any clinical procedure is carried out for purely cosmetic reasons.
>
>   Patients will want film star looks and expectations are high whenever cosmetic dentistry is carried out. Are you confident you can deliver patient's dreams? Because that is what you are doing.

The maintenance of function is imperative and a patient may be disappointed, angry or frustrated if there is any deterioration as a result of cosmetic treatment.

You're in this together . . .

Crown and bridge work must be of an exceptionally high standard and the difficult areas of tooth shade and mould shape to match existing teeth must be discussed at the chair side with the patient and, when possible, with a technician who must share responsibility in the fulfilment programme.

SECTION 4

DENTAL
LABORATORIES

HERE ARE THE BASICS

 Give this lot some thought!
The regulations you need, for a little light bedtime reading are:

- The Medical Devices Directive 93/42/EEC
- The Medical Devices Regulations 1994 S.I. No 3017

If they don't send you to sleep, nothing will!

You rely on the dental laboratory to provide timely and good quality prosthetic equipment. Your reputation can, on occasion, depend on the work provided by the laboratory. Ever found yourself juggling the competing pressures of standards and cost? In the current environment of the NHS this is not easy. However, you cut corners at your peril.

Are you happy with the laboratory's standard of work? Don't compromise, at the end of the day it is your reputation at stake. Whoever heard a patient say they got a great new look from a laboratory . . . ?

 Make a Note

Laboratory staff are not clairvoyant and instructions to them must be explicit in order to ensure that you get what you want and it is made from the materials you want.

If it is NHS work make it crystal clear to the lab. Where regulation dictates particular conditions (for example the amount of fine gold in a restoration), don't assume that the laboratory will comply with it.

STANDARDS

A number of standards apply to dental laboratories. The *Dental Laboratories Association* applies the *Dental Appliance Manufacturers Audit Scheme (DAMAS)*. Dentists may use DAMAS as the yardstick to assess the laboratory they work with. The full document may be obtained from the DLA.

It is reasonable for you to expect the appliance you ordered to meet your requirements and be fit for its purpose.

The dentist should be happy that the approach of the laboratory is satisfactorily audited and that audit trails are available. Accountability is paramount throughout the manufacturing process.

The manufacturer must be able to demonstrate that the appliance was made to the requirements stated by the dentist.

A copy of all work sheets, prescriptions and lab tickets should be retained in case of disagreement and should be legible. Amendments to work requirements must be recorded, authorised by the laboratory and dated. The laboratory should agree with the dentist the nature of materials required to provide a prosthesis of the required standard.

The laboratory must ensure that the staff employed are competent for the roles that they undertake. The laboratory should be able to provide information on the staff to confirm that they are suitably qualified.

Plus:

> **Make a Note**
>
> The dental appliance manufacturer must be registered with the Medical Devices Agency and be able to prove the registration. The only document that lists such laboratories is the DLA yearbook (information available from DAMAS – 0115 948 2400).

- the laboratory should ensure that training programmes exist for staff and that they are competent to carry out the tasks allocated to them
- the laboratory should be able to demonstrate a maintenance schedule and provide maintenance data if required
- the final product from the laboratory should receive a final inspection and quality control from a competent person.

. . . and just one or two more things, to plant the seeds of insomnia:

- the laboratory should have procedures for ensuring the appliances arrive in good condition
- the laboratory should ensure that suitable records of work undertaken, personnel involved, materials used and dates are maintained. The records should be kept for five years. Appliances should be suitably labelled.
- the laboratory should send out an invoice or label with each returned finished dental appliance. The label should state that the appliance is custom made for the patient. There should be a statement of work completed together with information on outstanding payments sent out at an agreed frequency (generally monthly).

You'll know you've got a good lab, if it:

- has a complaints procedure with agreed timescales. Corrective action should be reviewed by laboratory quality managers to ensure it is effective.
- has suitable insurance if appliances are sent through the post, unless you have alternative arrangements.

Make sure completed work is suitably handled, properly identified, packaged, stored, preserved and delivered to the surgery.

Have you got an enquiry line number to check on the progress of work at the lab? That way, when Mrs Chuffington-Smythe rings up about her new gnashers you'll be able to find out what's happening!

Sounds simple but make sure you can identify the patients for whom work has been carried out and

 Hazard Warning

There should be a system for discussing the laboratory's requirements in respect of the nature and standard of impressions, etc. This should be constructive, try to avoid it degenerating into a punch-up. Sort out what you want at contract review stage.

Dental material standards published by the British Standards Institution should be on your reading list – sorry, but it's important!

 Hazard Warning

Hydrocolloid impressions should not be sent through the post. They should be cast the same day either at the practice or after collection by the laboratory. If despatched to a laboratory the dentist should ensure that the impression is moist (wrapped in wet paper or in a humidor) until cast. It's a good idea to write the name of the patient in indelible pencil on the impression.

what charges are being made. In a busy practice it's easy to get into a muddle.

And, by the way, sort out an agreed complaints procedure to manage patient complaints and cases of appliance nonconformity. Be clear whose responsibility it is if appliances are lost in transit.

Have <u>you</u> got it right?

It's not all one-way traffic. You will be placing heavy demands on the lab. Make sure the materials you send are up-to-scratch. Be prepared to acknowledge and respect technical advice. Find out what you don't know, have a look at relevant ISO material standards and recognise your limitations.

Finally, labs can't work for fresh air and you get better service if you are a good customer and that includes paying your bills on time!

Using a laboratory meeting DAMAS standards? Here's what you can expect:

- that the laboratory complies with current legislation
- that the laboratory has documented processes and procedures including a complaints procedure
- that the laboratory undertakes regular internal audits and an annual independent external audit
- that the laboratory has a regular review of requirements
- that the laboratory provides advisory support as necessary.

The unified DAMAS standard may assist the dentist in reducing any technical risks to which he or she may be exposed. Makes sense to ensure that the laboratory providing the technical work meets the DAMAS or equivalent standard.

CHECK OUT YOUR DENTAL LABORATORY SERVICES

Yes

Done

On the way

By when?

- Do you know what you really want and does the lab give it to you?
- Do you have a system for ensuring that the instructions to the dental laboratory are explicit and include sufficient detail to enable the laboratory to meet the dentist's requirements?
- Does the laboratory comply with the requirements of the Medical Devices Directive and the Medical Devices Regulations?
- Do you have access to the audits that the laboratory undertakes of its own activities?
- Do you use dental impression materials and techniques of an adequate standard?
- Are you satisfied that the laboratory staff are trained to a satisfactory standard and that they have a continuing education programme?
- Are you satisfied that the laboratory uses properly maintained equipment of satisfactory standard and that the prostheses and environment is adequately cleaned?
- Do you have satisfactory arrangements for transporting and collecting technical work?

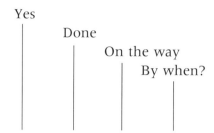

Yes
Done
On the way
By when?

- Do you have satisfactory arrangements for insuring technical work that is lost in the post?
- Do you receive satisfactory invoices allowing identification of the patient and a clear note of the charge made for the work?
- Is there a complaints procedure if the dentist or the patient is dissatisfied?
- Is there a mechanism for the laboratory to discuss the materials sent by the dentist if the technician does not feel able to undertake technical work of an adequate standard?
- Are you familiar with dental materials standards?
- Are laboratory accounts paid promptly?

DENTAL LABORATORY SERVICES CHECKLIST

Check!

Does the laboratory check in all cases that:

- the laboratory order is correctly followed
- all hydrocolloid impressions are collected and cast the same day
- the appliance fits the model accurately
- models occlude correctly

- models are clean and presentable
- the work has gone to the correct client?

With crown and bridgework does the laboratory check that:

- the item fits the die and model
- contact points are to requirements
- the porcelain has no faults or porosity
- the shade, glaze and form are correct
- that the precious metal content conforms to requirement or regulation
- metalwork has been correctly polished?

With orthodontic work does the laboratory check:

- all functional appliances on the articulator
- acrylic work for processing faults
- wires, screws and springs for damage, alignment and function
- acrylic and wire has been correctly polished?

With prosthetic work does the laboratory check:

- acrylic for porosity, movement of teeth, inclusion of foreign bodies
- that the acrylic has been properly polymerised
- the fitting surfaces for rough or sharp points
- the position of the post dam
- the correct depth of flanges and that there is correct muscle trimming
- acrylic has been polished
- there are no plaster traces?

With chrome cobalt work does the laboratory check:

- design is correct according to instructions
- there are no pointed or sharp edges
- acrylic retention is well applied and properly processed
- the chrome surfaces for casting faults
- that the metal is free from likely allergens such as nickel

- that a high lustre polish has been applied
- that it is free from investment and carbon inclusions?

Does the laboratory:

- discuss with the dentist at the review of requirements any perceived deficiencies in the clinical quality of impressions that might prevent the technician from constructing a satisfactory appliance
- believe that the dentist is approachable in respect of problems arising at the clinical/laboratory interface?

CLINICAL TREATMENT

AMALGAM RESTORATIONS

Did you know, amalgam has been used as a restorative material for 150 years. See, you've learned something! Worth the price of the book already!

But, for how much longer?

In recent times the use of amalgam has been repeatedly challenged from both within and outside the dental profession. The advantages and disadvantages of amalgam are well known but there is no reliable scientific data to suggest that amalgam either causes a general health hazard or that patients are hypersensitive to it.

At the present time, amalgam is regarded as a safe restorative material for patient use.

REMOVAL OF AMALGAM FILLINGS AT PATIENT'S REQUEST

If you've not been asked to do this, you will be! This is a recurring issue

There have been suggestions in the past that the removal of amalgam restorations and their replacement with other types of filling material may have an effect in the treatment of conditions such as multiple sclerosis and Alzheimer's disease.

There is no evidence to support this.

 Make a Note

Dentists should not recommend the replacement of amalgam restorations solely as a method of curing or alleviating diseases, infections or other medical conditions when it is not based on any clear scientific evidence – it's improper and unethical.

and most dentists are confronted at some time with a patient who asks for their amalgam fillings to be removed and replaced with what they describe as a non-toxic material. There are a number of indications for removing or replacing amalgam fillings.

These include:

- caries
- fracture of an existing restoration
- fracture of a tooth
- galvanic reactions
- cosmetic reasons under appropriate circumstances.

You should also know, that the consent of the patient for treatment is required. Consent may not be regarded as valid if there is not a clinical reason for replacing an amalgam restoration.

So, what do you do, when confronted with a patient hell-bent on having their amalgam restored when there is no defect? This is what:

- Explain to the patient that there is no requirement to replace the restoration.
- Advise the patient of the consequences of replacing an existing registration (e.g. loss of sound tooth structure).
- Indicate any risks or benefits of using a different replacement material.
- Make it clear that to replace any filling is not going to confer any improved medical benefit.

Still won't give up? The patient is insisting?

If the patient insists on having the filling replaced, the dentist must decide whether or not to comply with that request. There is no legal or ethical requirement to do so except in the very rare circumstance where it may be demonstrable that the patient actually has some sort of true allergy. Ultimately, and with the patient's consent based on a full understanding of the risks, benefits and consequences of changing a filling material, the dentist must exercise his own judgement about whether he feels content to do so.

Most commonly the reason for replacing a sound amalgam is that the patient requires cosmetic improvement. The dentist may well find such a reason acceptable and may progress subject to explanation and consent.

Expect the unexpected

During the course of dental treatment, from time to time you'll find the unexpected, e.g. a pulpal exposure or a fracture of tooth material. Don't worry, it isn't necessarily down to you for missing something. It is often the case that such findings could not be predicted either from clinical examination or radiographs.

What are you going to do?

- Don't leave the patient in the dark. Warn them, if the possibility actually exists however remote.
- Tell the patient what is going on.
- Explain how the proposed treatment will differ from the treatment plan already discussed as a result of your discovery.

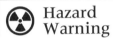 **Hazard Warning**
Try not to show surprise. It is more reassuring to the patient if you stay cool and avoid a, 'Wow! I never expected that!' . . . type of reaction!

- Keep the patient in the picture and they will not go home disappointed – they will, instead, think you are wonderful!

Restoration checklist

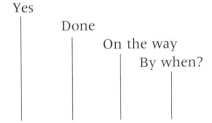

- Do you really recognise the toxicity of mercury and understand the potential consequences of inhalation, ingestion and absorption?
- Do you ensure mercury is dispensed using a funnel, gloves and a lipped tray?
- Do you have a mercury spillage kit?

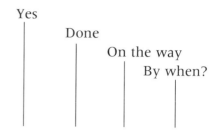

- Do you know where it is?
- Do you use pre-dispensed amalgam capsules?
- Do you use rubber dam where appropriate?
- Do you ensure that skin is thoroughly washed with soap and water and dried with a paper towel if in contact with mercury?
- Do you ensure that waste amalgam is stored in a recognised and labelled container?
- Do you ensure appropriate disposal of amalgam? What is it?
- Do you have a policy for managing patients who request removal or replacement of amalgam fillings?

PERIODONTAL DISEASE

In dental defence circles, they hear it all the time. Complaints or claims from patients in the area of periodontology.

There will be an allegation of failure to diagnose periodontal disease, failure to refer the patient to an appropriate specialist or failure to adequately treat the condition.

In most cases, this appears to be because the dentist is more preoccupied with examination of the hard tissues than of the soft tissues. Many examinations fail to include a full periodontal assessment including measurement of pocket depth.

FAILURE TO DIAGNOSE

The expectation of every patient is that the dentist knows what they are doing, is the next best thing to sliced bread and will do a full examination. Many patients never consider the prospect of periodontal disease or even understand the signifi-cance of it, even when their gums are bleeding or their teeth are loosening. So it's down to the dentist to do a bit of educashun!

In other words, make it clear to the patient the significance of periodontal disease and what is required to remedy any periodontal disease. Not only should the report contain the dentist's assessment of the periodontal condition but it should also contain a note of the ability of the patient to maintain oral hygiene.

A note:

 Make a Note

The dental record should include a specific note about the condition of the periodontium and the X-ray report should also indicate any areas of bone loss or other consequences resulting from periodontal disease.

Making decent notes and telling the patient what's going on is the best defence against a claim for alleged failures on the part of the dentist.

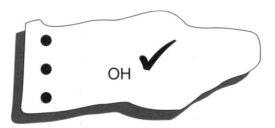

. . . . won't do!

Would you believe it? Some patients don't brush their teeth! There is often evidence that patients either fail altogether to brush their teeth, brush only parts of the teeth or cause damage to hard tissues and periodontal tissues as a result of inappropriate brushing of the teeth. What could their mothers have been thinking of?

Be sure to note these shortcomings in the dental record. To have noted these features indicates that the dentist is aware of the general clinical state of the patient.

Got a patient with periodontal disease? Be sure that:

- the clinical condition is fully documented
- the state of oral hygiene is fully documented
- the state of the periodontium and consequences of not treating it are explained to the patient
- the consequences of not undertaking the periodontal treatment are fully explained to the patient
- the patient is notified if they fail to complete periodontal treatment that, to do so could result in further chronic damage
- allow the patient to make a decision about whether they wish periodontal disease, particularly advanced disease, to be treated by the general practitioner or referred to a specialist. The patient may choose not to have the treatment at all (some patients are aware of the extremely poor prognosis and impending tooth loss). If this is the case ensure that it is **fully** documented in the notes.

CARRYING OUT A BASIC PERIODONTAL EXAMINATION (BPE)

- Examine the periodontium with a periodontal probe.
- Check the gingival crevice on all aspects of the tooth.
- Record the highest score in each sextant.

Scoring system:

0   Healthy gingival tissue.
1   Entire coloured band visible, no calculus, bleeding with probing.
2   As 1 but with calculus or defective margin.
3   Part of coloured band visible when probe is inserted into pocket (3.5–5.5 mm).
4   Entire coloured band disappears when probe inserted into pocket (5.5 mm +).
*   Total attachment loss of more than 7 mm.

PERIODONTOLOGY CHECKLIST

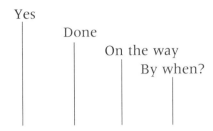

Yes
   Done
      On the way
         By when?

- Does the dentist have full periodontal charting for all patients?
- Does the dentist carry out a basic periodontal examination on every patient?
- Does the dentist repeat the BPE annually?
- Does the charting include history of all previous periodontal therapy including root planing and surgical treatment?

Does the dentist record the following:

- Assessment of oral hygiene
- Plaque scores
- Mobility
- Bleeding
- Probe depth chart
- Can the dentist identify the need for procedures such as grading and has this been documented?
- Does the dentist maintain the periodontal record and discuss it with the patient?
- Does the dentist refer periodontal patients when appropriate?
- Does the dentist record the reason for referral on the patient record card?
- Does the dentist use the specialist for a second opinion in respect of a treatment plan where the patient does not feel confident?

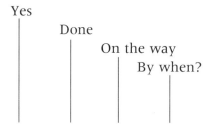

Yes

Done

On the way

By when?

- Does the dentist consult colleagues within the same practice when he feels uncertain about the management of periodontal disease?
- Does the dentist continually review periodontal disease and consider referral when the patient fails to respond to treatment?
- Does the dentist check recall charting against the baseline charting of the first visit to determine whether the patient's condition has deteriorated, stabilised or improved?
- Does the dentist recall patients for periodontal therapy in a timely and efficient manner?
- Does the dentist have a protocol for use by the staff to ensure that patients do not fail to attend for regular periodontal therapy?

ENDODONTICS

Every dentist has tales of distorted roots, blocked canals, apices that were impossible to seal and stories of broken reamers and files. So, it won't come as a surprise to learn that endodontic therapy is a cause of many claims for negligence.

Such joys include:

- failure to diagnose pulpal disease or identify a pulpal exposure
- failure to treat an established necrotic pulp
- failure to successfully manage a root canal therapy
- unnecessary root canal therapy.

Before embarking on endodontic treatment, it is important to fully assess the tooth both clinically and using radiographs so that teeth that may be impossible to adequately treat can be identified and the patient either warned or referred to a specialist more able to undertake the therapy. Such teeth are those with sclerotic canals and canal systems of unusual or dichotomous morphology.

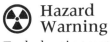 **Hazard Warning**

Endodontic treatment is very risky and a full explanation of the difficulties should be given to the patient at the outset.

You need to ask yourself, is the patient sufficiently compliant to undertake root canal therapy. The root canal treatment may require a number of visits and other treatment and clearly it is very dodgy to set out on such a treatment if it is likely to be left unfinished.

 Make a Note

It is important to remember that a patient may be referred at any stage during a root canal treatment. If you encounter particular difficulties and you feel that your degree of skill is such that you cannot resolve those difficulties, it is better to advise the patient of the changed circumstances and to direct the patient to a specialist. Don't be brave!

RUBBER DAM

Every dental student is taught how to use rubber dam during endodontic treatment. Can you remember your training? It is regarded by the dental schools as the minimum standard of care to:

- protect the patient
- maintain a dry environment
- prevent the accidental leakage of chemicals used in the therapy.

Occasionally, it may be that it is not possible to use a rubber dam because of the clinical state of the teeth, patient distress or other factors. In such circumstances, it is important to ensure that

 Hazard Warning

If, during the course of a root canal treatment where a patient does not have a rubber dam, chemicals or instruments are either swallowed or aspirated, a claim may be difficult to defend. It is up to the dentist in those circumstances to demonstrate the availability of an equally effective method of protecting the patient against such an event.

some sort of barrier is placed between the tooth and the back of the throat to minimise the potential risk of loss of a dropped instrument.

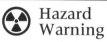 **Hazard Warning**

Even with the rubber dam in place, be sure to check it regularly to ensure that it has not become breached or that chemicals used during root canal therapy have not tracked between rubber dam and skin and caused chemical burns.

BROKEN INSTRUMENTS

During the course of endodontics, there is a risk that a reamer or a file may break in the root canal. Want to try to avoid it happening to you? Do this:

- Mandatory pre-operative radiographs to identify any root canal morphology which might pre-dispose to instrument breakage and also to enable measurement of the length of the root.
- Files, reamers and broaches should be checked to ensure that there is no evidence of damage.
- Instruments that have any visible defect including being bent or having part of a tip missing should be discarded.
- Filing and reaming techniques during endodontic work should be performed correctly and, if rotary reamers are employed, an endodontic hand piece should be used.
- Take radiographs during the course of endodontic treatment to confirm progress as required.
- Ensure that the instrument is of the correct working length before inserting it in the tooth.
- Irrigate the tooth frequently with standard irrigating solution.

 Make a Note

Still got a problem? Despite taking all the precautions, occasionally a root canal instrument may break. Don't worry, it is not necessarily negligent provided that you have taken suitable precautions beforehand and had followed an appropriate procedure.

If you do discover that an instrument has broken:

- Tell the patient immediately that the tip of an instrument has broken *(some authorities suggest it is more appropriate to describe the tip of the instrument having separated but this may be regarded as misleading).*
- Explain to the patient what modified treatment the dentist will now institute.
- Attempt to remove the piece of broken instrument from the tooth using an accepted technique. Try not to push the piece of broken instrument further into the tooth.
- If it is possible to remove the broken piece, measure it with the remainder of the instrument to ensure that the whole of the fragment has been removed. In addition it should be verified radiographically.
- If successfully removed, the broken instrument together with the fragment should be shown to the patient so that the patient is aware that it has been successfully retrieved.
- Make sure that the incident is documented in the record.
- If the fractured piece of reamer cannot be retrieved, the dentist should immediately consider referral to an endodontic specialist for evaluation, and advice or treatment. The referral letter should explain the events and give details of the nature of the instrument fragment left in the root canal.
- If the dentist decides, in consultation with the patient, not to refer, then the dentist should attempt to complete the root canal therapy by obturation of the canal up to and around the fragment as well as possible. The approach should be fully explained to the patient and the tooth should be regularly monitored at each recall to ensure that the outcome remains satisfactory.

If, following an attempt to restore the root canal with the fragment in place, the outcome is unsatisfactory, the dentist should refer the patient to an endodontist or an oral surgeon for evaluation for retrieval of the fragment or for apicectomy and retrograde root filling.

 Make a Note

The golden rule – again! At all times, it is important to document the events.

ENDODONTICS CHECKLIST

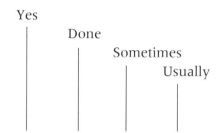

Yes

Done

Sometimes

Usually

- Only undertake root canal therapy for cases within your area of clinical expertise.
- Always have a pre-operative radiograph showing the entire root structure and the periapical area prior to initiating endodontic therapy.
- Take steps to confirm the correct tooth before creating an endodontic access.
- Only perform endodontic therapy on a tooth for which you have consent from the patient.
- Verify the root canal length by using a suitable radiographic technique.
- Verify the endodontic result with a radiograph of the filled canals. Is the X-ray dated and retained?
- Provide clear instructions to the patient about what symptoms may be expected and, in the event of the development of symptoms, what the patient should do both in hours and out-of-hours.
- Retain all root canal X-rays including those taken before, during and after the procedure.
- Adopt best practice of contacting a patient seven to ten days after root canal treatment to ensure that there have been no complications.
- Are the root canal instruments (reamers and files) replaced at regular intervals?

CROWN AND BRIDGE

No not the pub . . .

Is this the most difficult part of your work? The experts say it is.

Not only are there complex practical considerations, but there is a fine balance to be struck between the perception by the patient and the dentist of what constitutes satisfactory aesthetics. In other words how you look at a nice smile. Many claims arise as a result of bridge work which is not defective in some way but where the appearance has failed to meet patient expectations.

Commonly, crown and bridge work may fail because prepared teeth may fracture following the fitting of a crown or bridge because the tooth was over prepared. Insufficient tooth substance remains to bear the strains imposed upon it by the new crown or bridge, particularly if there is any element of malocclusion.

When preparing a crown or bridge, it is important to ensure that there is sufficient clinical crown height to support and retain the restoration. It is often tempting to try to get away with insufficient tooth rather than to undertake the necessary root canal therapy or thimble preparation. Whether or not the patient is keen to have the additional treatment to achieve a satisfactory outcome, it is certain that the patient will be dissatisfied if the crown is not suitably retained following fitting.

It is important that the dentist is not pressed into providing a design of crown or bridge preparation with which he or she does not feel confident. Both the dentist and the patient will have difficulties if such an approach is adopted.

Crown and bridge work may fail when such restorations are provided in the mouth of a patient with a poor periodontium. Indeed it may be the pre-existence of periodontal disease which has resulted in loss of teeth in the first place and the necessity for cosmetic or functional restorations.

 Make a Note

If, during the course of preparation, it becomes apparent that there may be insufficient substance to ensure that a strong crown or bridge can be fitted, the patient should be immediately informed and should be advised of any necessary adaptation in order to ensure that the problem can be remedied. And, remember the golden rule – make a note in the patient record.

In this event you should:

- ensure that the patient is fully informed of the periodontal condition and the fact that crown or bridge work is unlikely to succeed
- refuse to proceed if you suspect that any crown or bridge will have only a limited life because of the quality of the underlying support
- propose a programme of care that involves improving the periodontal state before embarking on complex and expensive restoration.

How common is this? The patient pitches up with a fractured incisor and the periodontal condition is poor. You'd probably advise extraction and restoration using a removable appliance. The patient screams they don't want a tooth in a jar and they want a nice crown – thank you very much!
What can be done?

- The situation should be made explicitly clear to the patient.
- Any decision should be made in the light of the condition of all the remaining teeth, particularly if the periodontal disease is more generalised or if other teeth have already been lost.
- If, having considered the overall clinical condition, best practice and the patient's wishes, you decide to proceed, then you should institute an immediate programme of patient education and periodontal treatment to stabilise and improve the periodontal state. Where possible a temporary restoration can be supplied while work on the periodontal condition proceeds. You may inform the patient that permanent restoration of the tooth will not begin until some periodontal parameters have been met. In other words clean your gob up!
- You should ensure that you have clear patient consent for the programme proposed.
- Don't be a hero and try taking on therapy that is destined to fail. Though in the short term you may be applauded by the patient, support and enthusiasm will soon give way to anger and opposition if the outcome is unsatisfactory.

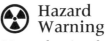 **Hazard Warning**

Many dentists feel that it is unfair that they may be held responsible for the patient's inability to understand the nature of treatment or to comply with the requirements. However, dentists do have a duty of care and they are at risk of being held liable in the event of failure. Patients are held less liable for being irresponsible than dentists!

- As with other forms of treatment, you cannot be obliged to undertake any treatment that you consider to be inappropriate or unacceptable. It is unethical to do so. In these circumstances, you should refuse and, if necessary, the patient can seek the advice of another dentist.

CROWN AND BRIDGE CHECKLIST

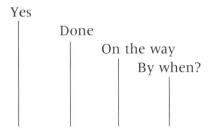

Yes

Done

On the way

By when?

- Are you a hero or do you select only those crown and bridge projects that are within your area of clinical expertise?
- Refer any appropriate case to a restorative specialist.
- Provide a written treatment plan for all restorative cases.
- Have a pre-operative radiograph showing the entire root structure and the periapical area prior to preparing the tooth.
- Carefully assess the periodontal and periapical status of the tooth or teeth prior to preparation.
- Document all X-ray results.
- Document the discussion with the patient and the consent that is agreed.
- Resist restoring those teeth with a very unfavourable or hopeless prognosis.
- Double check the tooth before starting work.

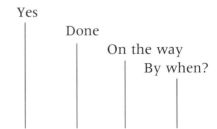

Yes
| Done
| | On the way
| | | By when?

- Provide clear instructions, either written or verbal, to patients following preparations for crowns and bridges, including any symptoms which the patient might experience and does the patient know how to contact you both in hours and out of hours should problems arise?
- Contact the patient a few days after completing crown and bridge work in order to check that all is well.
- Mention the consequences of exposure and loss of tooth vitality.

ORAL SURGERY

Be clear about this:

If you do carry out oral surgery and it is subsequently the subject of a claim for negligence, you may well find that, if the procedure you have attempted may be considered to be complex, your performance is measured against that of an ordinarily skilled oral surgeon rather than an ordinarily skilled dental practitioner.

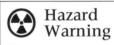 **Hazard Warning**

Never, never, never attempt an oral surgical procedure for which you are insufficiently experienced or competent.

Sound like basic advice? It is. But you'd never guess the number of times the advice is ignored and the dentist gets into trouble.

  Have a think before you start.

Prior to discussion with the patient, always consider all the possible complications which may arise and make a personal decision about whether the procedure should be attempted.

If, when you've had a 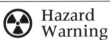 you decide to proceed, make sure you explain in detail to the patient what's involved, the consequences of providing it in the surgery and any risks or benefits of undertaking it in the practice. It may also be wise to give the patient the option of having the treatment carried out in the hospital.

Oral surgery procedures where complications are foreseeable include:

- the extraction of impacted teeth
- the extraction of teeth with divergent roots
- the extraction of teeth with unusually long or bulbous roots
- the extraction of ankylosed teeth
- the extraction of teeth with roots which impinge upon one of the sinuses or on the inferior dental canal
- the surgical treatment of patients who are very nervous or have physical or mental disability which might make the procedure very difficult or impossible in a general practice setting
- surgical procedures in patients who are unreliable or uncooperative and who may not return for follow-up appointments
- surgical treatment for those patients with medical conditions which may predispose to surgical complications.

Extraction of an incorrect tooth occurs surprisingly frequently and mainly for these 'popular' reasons:

- lack of concentration on the part of the dentist
- lack of adequate communication between the patient and the dentist
- charting anomaly, e.g. two molar teeth which may be charted as six and seven or seven and eight.

> **⚠ Hazard Warning**
>
> Extraction of the wrong tooth? Best avoided. Remember:
>
> CHECK TWICE,
> EXTRACT ONCE!

- If the tooth has a particular characteristic which identified it, note it to minimise confusion when it is extracted.
- Chart two standing molars as 68 rather than 67 or 78.
- Safety should take precedence over anatomical accuracy.

If it's got to come out:

- Make a clear note of the reason for the extraction. This should include patient complaints, clinical findings (percussion mobility, sensitivity, etc.).
- Give a clear indication of why you support the recommendation to extract.
- If the patient is referred to another dentist for the extraction, it is important to double check and confirm with the patient which tooth is to be extracted before it is written in a letter of referral.
- There should normally be a radiograph of the tooth to be extracted and it may be wise to mark it on the X-ray to minimise risk of error.
- Always state on the appointment which tooth or teeth is or are to be extracted rather than simply writing extractions. Such a note provides a further safeguard.

. . . and when it gets complicated:

Expect the unexpected, it's bound to happen to you. For example a fracture of a tooth root or unexpected bleeding. Ever happened to you? What emotions did you experience?

- Stress
- Anxiety
- Anger
- Harassment.

. . . or even panic. Don't worry, you're not the first. Stay cool and here's what you do:

- Assess whether the procedure, including any possible foreseeable complication, falls within your skill level. **If not, a patient should be referred**.
- If there are any complications that the dentist would not be prepared to handle, the patient should be advised that, in the event of them occurring, the patient will be referred to a specialist. This reduces the element of surprise if a complication arises and referral becomes necessary. If the patient is concerned that this sort of situation may arise, it is probably expedient to refer the patient to a specialist anyway.
- **Make clear to the patient that you are not into heroic surgery. The problem will be sorted but not by you. That's smart. Bodging on isn't.**
- Make clear that the objective is to achieve the desired result with the least trauma and that the procedure will be pursued in that way.
- If a referral occurs in the middle of a procedure, you should have in place a policy for managing such a case. This might include arrangements to telephone a surgeon directly and a procedure for following up the patient after the treatment has been completed, i.e. enquiring directly of the patient how they are two to three days after the completion of the procedure and offering further support should they need it.

If a complication arises, particularly one that requires a referral, the dentist should have a policy in place in respect of charging the patient, whether private or NHS. It may well be expedient to waive any charges associated with untoward or undesirable effects.

POST-OPERATIVE COMPLICATIONS

Patients may suffer unpredictable post-operative complications. These may include things like dry socket or unexpected or recurrent bleeding.

Don't be shy and don't be secretive. Warn the patients what complications may arise, for example infection, bleeding, swelling, pain and anaesthesia or paraesthesia. It's a lot easier for them to cope with the expected. The unexpected brings its own level of anxiety. Advise any patient on whom you are undertaking a surgical procedure what is the usual routine for managing any complications. Advise them where and when they should go if symptoms arise, what would be required in general terms for management and how to contact the dentist both in and out of hours.

Don't treat post-operative complications casually. With bleeding and infection particularly, satisfy yourself that they are brought under control rather than simply offering telephone advice without reviewing the patient directly. If the patient attends the surgery it gives you a far better chance of making a correct diagnosis and prescribing correct treatment.

Don't take a chance – take a look!

 Make a Note

Even a simple complication, seemingly minor when explained on the telephone, should be treated as potentially serious and the patient should be asked to come to the practice.

POST-OPERATIVE CARE AND FOLLOW-UP

Get this right and you'll have:

- the opportunity to identify any unexpected consequences that may need further treatment
- an opportunity to learn of any problems, complaints or compliments (yes, they are not unheard of) they may offer
- an opportunity to strengthen a dentist/ patient relationship by showing interest and involvement in the care.

 Make a Note

How do your patients make contact if they have a problem? Put in place arrangements to ensure that, should complications arise from surgery, the patient is able to contact someone for advice or assistance.

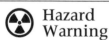 Hazard
Warning

Special care must be taken in respect of specimens excised for histological examination. It is vital that any biopsy sent from the practice should be recorded and it should be confirmed that the histological report is received back. It should be signed as having been read by the operator and arrangements should be made to ensure that the patient is informed of the result. Failure to do so, in the event of a malignancy, may have very serious consequences.

It is important to remember that in the event that the dentist is accused of some form of negligent act as a consequence of surgical complications, general dental practitioners undertaking surgical procedures beyond those that would normally be associated with general dental practice will be measured against the standards of an oral surgeon with the degree of skill that such a procedure implies.

The message is, don't over-extend your practice.

SURGICAL CHECKLIST

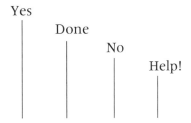

Yes

Done

No

Help!

- Select cases within your clinical expertise.
- Refer patients when appropriate.
- Always have a pre-operative radiograph showing the entire root structure prior to extraction when any potential difficulty may be perceived or expected.
- Verify that the correct tooth is extracted.
- Only extract teeth when you have consent.
- Provide clear oral or written instructions about the method by which post-operative complications will be managed.
- Make clear to the patient how the dentist should be contacted both in and out of hours in the event of complications arising.
- Make a courtesy call to the patient following surgery by way of follow-up.
- Insist that every patient re-attends for at least one follow-up appointment following surgery.
- Document all pre-operative, intra-operative and post-operative findings and details in the dental record.

PROSTHETICS

Is there a dentist alive without a story of denture failure? Patients think they're wearing someone else's teeth. They don't like the smile, they can't get used to using them.

This is all very frustrating to patients who expected an easy transition, especially when a friend or relative had an easy experience when he or she was first provided with a denture.

Be prepared. In general, patients blame the dentist for denture failures rather than themselves. Why not? That's why you're paid all this money!

For the average dental practitioner, the prospect of making a denture for a patient with a minimal ridge or with flaccid musculature, is a daunting task which, in a number of cases, is doomed to failure from the outset.

When you undertake removable prosthetic work for a patient, try to minimise the possibility of complications with these six steps:

- Try to assess patient expectations beforehand.
- Explain to the patient the problems associated with the denture and emphasise the difficulties that the patient might experience.
- Make clear to the patient that dentures replace only the teeth and that, although they may produce some facial cosmetic improvement by providing support for facial soft tissues, they cannot in any way improve general facial appearance.
- Make clear to the patient that there may be some time when the patient may be without dentures.
- Make clear to the patient that the dentures may not be ideal at first insertion and that adjustments may be required. If the dentist suspects that the patient has expectations that cannot be met, then make it clear and think about declining to provide the treatment.
- Document on the patient's records any particular areas of concern and the reasons why any patient is declined for treatment when expectations are impossible to meet.

During the preparation of dentures, there is often scope for misunderstanding to arise between you and the patient.

Entries like these in the dental record are not good enough:

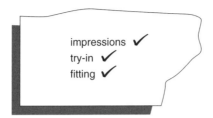

impressions ✓
try-in ✓
fitting ✓

Any claim against a dentist is easier to defend if the patient's agreement has been obtained and documented at each stage during the construction of the dentures.

Immediate dentures may provide a particular problem. Make sure the patient understands, quite clearly, that immediate dentures cannot accurately fit the mouth even at the time of insertion and that, as bone is resorbed they rapidly become looser.

During the stress of treatment patients may forget or misconstrue elements of your explanation. Better to give them a written sheet making clear that immediate dentures, though providing a cosmetic substitute, do not fulfil the other criteria of a satisfactory denture and are only a temporary substitute.

> **Make a Note**
>
> Make it clear to patients at the outset that, at the least, it is likely that it will be necessary to reline the dentures within a short period of time and that a new set of dentures, with consequent extra cost and time commitments, may be required within six months or so.

PROSTHETICS CHECKLIST

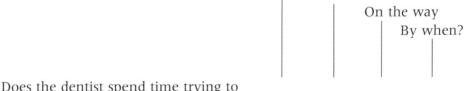

	Yes	Done	On the way	By when?
• Does the dentist spend time trying to establish the patient's expectations of the dentures and record any specific factors or anticipated problems?				
• Does the dentist emphasise the difficulties associated with dentures?				
• Does the dentist make clear that dentures cannot improve general facial appearance?				

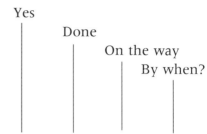

Yes
 Done
  On the way
   By when?

- Does the dentist explain the complications of immediate dentures and indicate the events following fitting?
- Does the dentist provide a leaflet about immediate dentures?
- Does the dentist record in detail the factors associated with each stage of denture construction, e.g. tooth shade, mould, patient wishes, etc.?
- Does the dentist spend time at the try-in stage to discuss tooth mould, shade and setting?
- Does the dentist agree to see the patient for any adjustments within 24 hours of fitting a new denture?

PAEDODONTICS AND ORTHODONTICS

Got kids? Then you'll know that paediatric dentistry involves a complex interaction between the child, the parent and the dentist.

This is not easy and certainly not for everyone. There are special skills needed. Because you are good with your own kids, or your sister's kids, or the kids next door that doesn't necessarily mean you'll be good will every kid and certainly not the ones who have toothache or who are frightened stiff by the thought of a visit to the dentist.

It is often a cause of complaint that children are not 'handled' by dentists in a way that is approved by the parents. Eliminate or minimise those problems by spending time with the parent beforehand explaining how the child will be managed and seeking the parent's consent for the management programme proposed.

It is often helpful to try to engage the assistance of the parent in managing the child. To provide the parent with a seat near the child may be more effective than keeping the parent at a significant distance. If, having outlined the way in which you propose to treat the child, the parent disagrees, then think hard about what you want to do. Declining treatment might be the best option. Don't be swayed by the parents perceptions. Offer to do what is right for the child in a way that you are comfortable with. Anything else is a disaster waiting to happen.

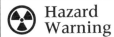 **Hazard Warning**

Dentists undertaking paedodontics need to consider the design of the surgery:

- safety
- entertainment
- parental access
- noise control.

Orthodontic treatment should only be provided by dentists who are entirely competent to undertake it. In no area of treatment is a full pre-treatment assessment and an agreed written treatment plan more important. The treatment plan should be talked through with the parents and the child before any orthodontic treatment is embarked on and, where possible, a signed consent should be obtained.

In the event that the patient moves house during a course of orthodontic treatment, a copy of the treatment plan can then go to the new orthodontist for the treatment to be continued.

Sometimes, when a patient does change orthodontists, the new orthodontist does not agree with the approach of the former orthodontist. For that reason, in addition, a fully-documented and agreed programme is very important.

If you inherit a patient halfway through treatment and you're not happy with the approach, do this:

- Contact the first orthodontist to discuss the case and understand why the orthodontist adopted the approach.
- Consider whether the original orthodontist approach, though at variance with the approach of the second orthodontist, may in fact produce an acceptable outcome without the need for change.
- If a change is required, explain the alteration with tact and diplomacy.

> ☢ Hazard
> Warning
>
> Orthodontics is unusual in that it is not generally possible to suspend treatment without the development of adverse effects. This factor, combined with the fact that orthodontics takes a significant time, may have consequences if a child's parents are separated or divorced.
>
> It may be that the child is brought by different parents for orthodontic consultations at different times and, if the parental split is acrimonious, the individual parents may adopt different perspectives in respect of the form in which the treatment is provided.
>
> Don't get trapped between two opinions. Provide two copies of ongoing treatment plans, one to each parent, at the onset of treatment with further information provided to both parents as the treatment progresses.
>
> If a parental dispute makes the continuance of orthodontic treatment impossible, the dentist should write to both parents before considering giving up. The letter should contain information about the consequences of stopping treatment, the difficulties and costs associated with restarting it, the need for additional visits on the part of the child if more treatment is required. When this sort of problem arises, make sure that all parental discussions are documented and, if possible, witnessed.

GILLICK COMPETENCE

Remember that? Have a look at p. 18 – oh, don't bother, here it is again.

>
>
> Children over sixteen are regarded as adult and enjoy the same rights of consent as adults.
>
> Children under the age of sixteen have the right to make their own decision about consent provided they have sufficient maturity to understand the nature of the matter requiring a decision. 'Gillick competence' imparts the notion of having sufficient maturity and intelligence to fully understand what is proposed and its consequences in order to give consent.
>
> Assessment of 'Gillick competence' is a matter of clinical judgement for the dentist and recognises the right of self-determination of a young person and acknowledges that parental rights over children are dwindling and can be over-ridden.

> The Gillick case occurred in 1985 (*Gillick v West Norfolk and Wisbech Area Health Authority*). Mrs Victoria Gillick sought to prevent contraception being prescribed for her daughter(s) under the age of 16 without her knowledge. The consequences of the judgement have been rolled out across all areas of investigation and treatment in medicine and dentistry.
>
> In Scotland the issue is governed by the Age of Legal Capacity (Scotland) Act 1991. It is a statutory approach to the common law situation that exists in England and Wales.

CHILDREN'S DENTISTRY CHECKLIST

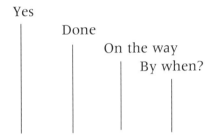

Yes

Done

On the way

By when?

- Have a clear plan for dealing with children.
- Have the necessary competence.
- Produce a detailed orthodontic treatment plan.
- Ensure that the parents of the child (when appropriate) understand fully the reason and nature of every step in the orthodontic process.
- In the event of a parental dispute, have a policy for managing the problem with minimal damage to the child or the treatment.
- Understand Gillick competence.

IMPLANTS

With an increase in popularity, so has come an increase in claims against dentists about their use of implants. And, implants tend to be more costly

than other forms of dental claim because of the extensive damage and the
difficulty of providing any sort of restoration when an implant has failed.
  Why do implants fail?

- The loss of significant amounts of bone which makes restoring the
  patient to a pre-implant state more difficult.
- Patient expectations of implant dentistry are often very high. This may
  be engendered by very positive marketing and media articles about
  the success of such implants. Advertising frequently claims that
  implants are 'far better' than dentures or bridge work. It is hardly
  surprising that patients feel very disappointed when they do not have
  the success.
- Implant surgery, which is not available on the NHS, is far more
  expensive than other forms of dentistry. It therefore involves a much
  greater financial as well as personal commitment on the part of the
  patient. Failure, therefore, has much more profound consequences and
  patients will be much more keen to place blame on the practitioner and
  to seek retribution and recompense when the process fails.

PICKING WINNERS

Picking winners, or case selection, is a smart way to stay out of trouble. Only
cases with a good long term prognosis should be selected. Here are some
guidelines for picking winners:

- Systemic factors including overall health, diseases such as diabetes or
  bleeding disorders and systemic diseases which might compromise
  immunity or general health.
- Local factors including adequacy of bone, oral hygiene, state of the
  occlusion, morphology of the ridge, quality of the bone, sinus and nerve
  position where relevant, general periodontal status, and the distance
  between the proposed fixation sites.
- Other factors include the use of tobacco or alcohol, patient attitude,
  financial considerations and how reasonable the patient's expectations are.

If a patient is considered suitable for implants, then great care should be
taken in planning. There must be good communication between the
restorative dentist, the dental technician and the surgeon to ensure that
nothing can go wrong.

Radiographs and diagnostic models should be used to properly assess the implant site. The procedures adopted during the marking, preparation and insertion of the implant should meet the highest standards of modern accepted practice.

Claims for negligence in cases of implant insertion can arise due to:

- failure of the system
- infection
- loosening
- poor aesthetics
- poor occlusion.

. . . The last two can often be traced to inadequate case planning.

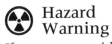 **Hazard Warning**

If you are providing implants be prepared to say 'no' to any candidate who is considered a poor risk.

If such a patient insists on having implants, the best risk management approach for the dentist is to refuse and suggest that they go elsewhere.

Failed implants are not only costly but may also be very damaging to a dentist's reputation in view of the high profile publicity that they may attract.

Good risk management is to identify any potential risk and to discuss it with the patient beforehand. A patient who is not fully informed of the risks and hazards of implant surgery is not in a position to have given adequate consent for the procedure to go ahead. These patients represent a claim waiting to happen.

PRESCRIPTIONS AND OTHER MEDICATION

When taking a medical history of any new patient or checking that no changes have arisen in the medical status of an existing patient, find out about and record any medication that they might be taking. It's simple enough – just ask!

A working knowledge of the nature and effects of medication and its impact on any dental procedure is important. In the event of an avoidable drug complication or inter-action, claiming ignorance of that contra-indication or interaction is a very poor defence.

There may also be circumstances where you will find it necessary to prescribe

A dentist may write a private prescription which may be cheaper than an NHS pre-scription from the patient's own GP. However, be careful about prescribing outside the area of your expertise.

medication for a patient. You may be asked to advise on buying some over-the-counter remedies. Often you will write a script for an analgesic, or antibiotic. Whether medication is advised or prescribed, obey the golden rule and note it in the dental records. Are you tired of that phrase, by now?

In the case of prescription drugs, the note should contain the name of the drug, the strength, the dose, the quantity of medication prescribed and the instructions for taking the medication. Don't use any abbreviations that are capable of misinterpretation. When writing the prescription itself, don't use annotation that is capable of being misunderstood by a pharmacist.

We've all had a laugh about doctors' disgusting handwriting. Even GPs are learning, clear writing makes for reliable records and safe scripts!

Although the pharmacist has, as part of his or her role, to check the medication and ensure that the prescription is correct, don't rely on them digging you out of a mess – mistakes do slip by.

Dentists may only write NHS prescriptions for those drugs that are included in the Dental Practitioner's Formulary. So, do you know which antibiotics are available to you, for the treatment of dental infections? In general, the Dental Practitioner's Formulary is adequate to meet almost any eventuality. However, on occasion, a patient may need a medication that falls outside the drugs available in the Dental Practitioner's Formulary. In that circumstance, speak to the patient's GP and ask for a prescription for the patient.

Details of the conversation should be, guess what? Yup, you're learning! Recorded in the dental record.

Be very careful when prescribing outside your area of expertise. If you see a patient who has an infection that is not related to the practice of dentistry, make an appropriate referral, usually to the patient's GP.

Don't be tempted to treat the problem yourself. Content yourself with being a dentist – at least for the time being!

 Make a Note

When prescribing for a patient, ensure that the patient understands what can be expected of the drug. The patient should not be given the impression that a drug will work instantly when, in reality, it may take two or three days to start to have an effect.

It is also important to inform the patient of any potential side effects or risks associated with the drug and advice on what to do should any complication arise.

Prescribing checklist

                                                        Yes
                                                          | Done
                                                          | | Got it
                                                          | | |
                                                          | | |

- Understand the prescriber has clinical responsibility for
  the use of the drug.
- Understand that, when using a drug, you should be
  aware of its indications, benefits, side-effects and
  contraindications.
- Understand that, if recommending an over-the-counter
  remedy, you may be asked to explain and justify the
  advice given if complications arise.
- Ensure that prescriptions have the following information:

  > Name (surname and one forename)
  > Address
  > Name of drug
  > Strength in milligrams
  > Quantity
  > Instructions about dosage and frequency
  > Signature and date in indelible ink.

- Understand the hazards of recommending or prescribing a
  drug with a therapeutic purpose outside dentistry.

Managing the dentist–patient relationship

Is everybody happy?

There's a lot more to being a dentist than being a dentist.

If you appear uncommunicative, arrogant, nervous, disinterested, or lacking in confidence, you will have a far more difficult task in establishing a rapport with a patient. This easily has a knock-on effect for discussions with the patient about the nature of their treatment.

A patient who feels at ease and confident in your ability is much more likely to be able to discuss concerns and requirements as well as the technical aspects of the provision of dental care.

Good relationships result in:

• greater agreement and compliance
• increased likelihood that the patient will actually be satisfied with the outcome of the work that is undertaken
• a reduced likelihood that the patient may complain or lodge a claim about the work which is provided.

. . . so, it's worth working at!

Managing 'risk' in the relationship – here are the basics:

• ensure that everything that you do is reasonable
• observe the common courtesies in terms of greetings and farewells
• observe the usual pleasantries by chatting during long periods where silence would otherwise occur
• treat the patient as intelligent but uninformed when explaining about proposed treatments and options.

 Make a Note

Remember the old saying:

'your friends don't sue you'.

Though not a cast-iron guarantee, it is often the case that a good relationship can overcome treatment difficulties or disappointments.

If the patient appears confused or lacking in understanding about a particular procedure, be patient, take time to explain it again and don't get irritated. If the treatment plan is complex, once it has been discussed suggest that the patient takes away the written treatment plan to think about and consider with friends or family and to return again to ask further questions before agreeing to and embarking on treatment.

Be friendly but not over friendly.

HEALTH AND SAFETY

INTRODUCTION

For most dental practices their biggest asset is their practice surgery. Increasingly practitioners are working from premises owned by health authorities or other outside bodies. Either way, the smart dentist is aware of health and safety requirements as they relate to issues ranging from the employment of staff to cross infection control procedures.

Not up to speed? Surely not! Well you're in luck because here is the dummies guide:

Under Section 2 of the Health and Safety at Work Act 1974, a dentist has certain responsibilities to all persons at work whether they are employers, employees or self-employed. Failure to act responsibly can lead to prosecution by the Health and Safety Executive. Who, incidentally, does not mess about!

The responsible employer (that means you) must provide and maintain a safe place of work, with safe equipment and procedures in place.

It's not all one way. Employees have responsibilities, too. They include the responsibility to have due regard for

. . . if you are a really sad person you'll probably already have read the relevant legislation. If not, you should at least have copies of this stuff and be on 'passing acquaintance' terms with it.

- Health and Safety at Work Act 1974
- Health and Safety Information for Employees Regulations 1989
- Management of Health and Safety at Work Regulations 1999

health and safety rules and procedures, and to report anything that could compromise this to the person in charge (that probably means you).

Health and safety legislation is becoming more risk-led. In plain English, that means there is a specific duty placed upon employers to assess the risks to their employees and others who may be affected by their work activities.

The requirement to assess risks may be general (Management of Health and Safety at Work Regulations 1999) or specific (COSHH Regulations).

Under health and safety law, an employer is required to display various things. Here's some stuff you've gotta do, or else:

- Display a health and safety poster. 'Health and Safety law – what you should know', in the practice to ensure compliance with the Health and Safety Information for Employees Regulations 1989.
- Display a current certificate of employer's liability.
- Display a written health and safety policy. This is a requirement of practices with five or more employees and it should be brought to the employee's attention.

Policy, policy? What the *&%% goes into that? Don't panic – here it is:

- A statement of the employer's commitment to providing a safe and healthy working environment.
- Details of safe working practices.
- Details of responsibilities for health and safety throughout the workplace.

The Health and Safety Executive is the statutory body responsible for enforcing the Health and Safety at Work Act and its inspectors have the power to inspect premises to ensure that they comply with the regulations and may ask to see the written Health and Safety policy statement.

 Make a Note

Got any youngsters working for you? Work experience, Saturday staff and such like?

The Health and Safety (Young Persons) Regulations 1997 were incorporated into the Management of Health and Safety at Work Regulations 1999, under which employers are required to carry out a risk assessment to young people (under age 18) in the workplace. When employing young people dentists should take into account their immaturity and inexperience, and provide appropriate training on practice procedures and health and safety issues.

. . . and they do! Not had a visit? You will have!

In practice, the local health authority regularly inspects dental surgeries and a health and safety assessment forms part of this procedure.

Just to be official, for a moment . . .

Dentists working within the NHS are required to permit these inspections as part of their terms of service (Para 33(4) of Part V of the NHS (General Dental Services) Regulations 1992). If the Health Authority has concerns regarding the condition of the premises, it may advise the HSE of this and the HSE has the power to enter the premises to investigate. If breaches of the legislation are identified the HSE Inspector can issue an improvement notice or a prohibition notice. Prosecution could also result in a fine of up to £20 000.

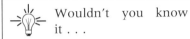 Wouldn't you know it . . .

The GDC also has a view on these matters and 'Maintaining Standards' has sections on dealing with cross-infection (Para 4.1) and disposal of clinical waste (Para 6.4).

Don't relax – there's more . . .

Six further sets of Health and Safety at Work Regulations came into force on 1 January 1993. They implement EC directives and update our existing law. They cover:

- general health and safety management
- work equipment safety
- manual handling of loads
- workplace conditions
- personal protective equipment
- display screen equipment.

Just in case you were confused, they clarify and make more explicit existing Health and Safety law.

Just for starters, here's the . . .

HEALTH AND SAFETY INTRODUCTORY CHECKLIST

It's a Yes or a No

* Do the premises comply with applicable local building codes and regulations?
* Do you have adequate public liability insurance to cover your premises?
* Is there a certificate of public liability insurance on display?

DUTIES TO STAFF

In other words, your duties as the employer . . .

All employers must ensure, so far as is reasonably practicable, the health, safety and welfare at work of all employees. This duty of care extends to patients and to self-employed contractors who may be on the premises.

As an employer a dentist must do a risk assessment of the practice in order to assess any potential hazards. This is a requirement of all employers.

Included within this risk assessment a dentist must do a risk assessment of all materials used within the practice. A court might well look at the cost of any preventive measures and weigh this against the risk of personal injury and likely severity.

All systems of work must be safe and without risk to health and this applies to all equipment used within a place of work. Equipment must be regularly maintained, renewed and serviced.

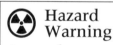 **Hazard Warning**

An employee could report a breach of the employer's statutory duty under the Act to the Health and Safety Executive, which could bring criminal charges.

The employee could further sue the employer for being in breach of this statutory duty as an employer or for negligence at common law.

Safe systems of work must be in place and used by all persons, e.g. arrangements for the safe disposal of waste and correct use of VDU equipment.

You must:

- provide a written policy statement on health and safety if you employ five or more staff
- provide and maintain safe equipment, appliances and systems of work
- assess all equipment and systems of work for risk
- initiate safe systems of work
- maintain the place of work, including the means of entrance and exit, in a safe condition
- provide a working environment for employees that is safe, without risk to health and with adequate facilities and arrangements for their welfare at work
- provide the necessary instruction, training and supervision to ensure health and safety
- arrange safe disposal of waste
- ensure that dangerous or potentially harmful substances or articles are handled and stored safely.

THE WRITTEN POLICY STATEMENT

Dentists who employ five or more staff must prepare a written statement of the practice's policy *'with respect to the health and safety'* of its employees. This must include details of the organisation and arrangements for carrying out this policy and the immediate action required by staff in respect of any accidents that occur.

Health and safety policy statements usually consist of three parts:

- a statement of intent which is a declaration of the employer's commitment to providing a safe and healthy workplace and environment
- details of responsibilities for health and safety throughout the workplace
- details of safe systems of work and safe working practices for all work activities.

 Make a Note

Although it is not necessary in a small practice to give everyone a copy of this written statement, it may be a jolly good idea!

The statement should also include the practice's policy on violence and infection control, and first aid arrangements.

DUTIES TO STAFF CHECKLIST

There's not a lot of options here, it's just got to be done;

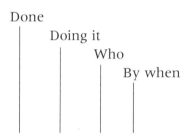

Done
   Doing it
      Who
         By when

- Does the dentist understand the duties to the staff?
- Does the dentist undertake a risk assessment of the potential hazards of the practice?
- Does the dentist review all the materials used within the practice?
- Is the dentist satisfied that all systems are safe and without risk to health?
- Does the dentist with more than five staff provide a written policy statement on health and safety?
- Does the dentist maintain the place of work in a safe condition?
- Does the dentist provide the necessary instruction, training and supervision to ensure health and safety?
- Does the dentist arrange the safe disposal of waste?
- Are potentially harmful substances handled and stored safely?
- Does the dentist in a small practice, though not required by law to do so, give everyone a written statement?

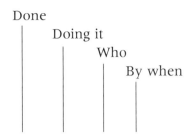

Done

Doing it

Who

By when

- Does the dentist strongly advise all staff to be immunised against diphtheria, tetanus, whooping cough, TB (BCG), rubella and hepatitis B?
- Does the dentist keep a staff immunisation log?
- Does the dentist ensure that any staff member refusing hepatitis B vaccine after explanation of risks and consequences signs a form to confirm that they have been advised?

PREMISES

Here's what the rules say:

Dentists, *'so far as is reasonably practicable as regards any place of work under [his or her] control'*, must ensure that the building is maintained in a safe condition, without risks to health. He or she must provide a safe means of entrance or exit for staff.

Here's a tricky bit:

. . . if the practice occupies a health centre under the direct control of a health authority, he or she can only do what is reasonable on his or her part, and any blame may ultimately lie with the health authority, e.g. any loose guttering which is the duty of the health authority to maintain under the terms of the licence, is the responsibility of the authority provided that the dentist had notified the authority (preferably in writing) of the danger. He or she would be exonerated if an accident occurred.

 Make a Note

Staff have a responsibility to report any risks to health and safety. If they do, be nice to them. They may save loadsa grief in the long run. Whatever it is, get it fixed, seen to, or sorted.

. . . so you're off the hook.

Similar conditions may arise when premises are rented from a private landlord. It may be advisable for you to have your lawyer take a good look at the licence or lease under which the premises are held. Have them clarify whose duty it is to maintain specific parts of the premises.

Beware . . .

A practice may not be exonerated of all responsibility for the safety of the premises, even if it does not own them. It may be held responsible for hazards such as highly polished and slippery floors and unsafe electrical flex. But if the dentist is responsible for maintaining the premises he or she must be concerned with other parts, including, for example, the condition of steps and stairways, floors and floor covering.

The Act also states that, as far as reasonably practicable, the employer must provide and maintain a working environment for employees which is without risk to health and with adequate provision for their general welfare. The wording appears to apply to more than just the physical environment of the employee. In this circumstance a practice would be well advised to consider whether there is an adequate rest-room, refreshment facilities and toilet and washing arrangements, etc. The extent to which this can be done depends on the practice's resources.

Alterations to existing buildings, or the building of new premises, should take account of health and safety and the security aspects of general practice. Wide doorways, grab rails and ramps and as few steps as possible. Think of those in wheelchairs, parents with small children, the elderly and the infirm and, to a certain extent, other users of the building.

Dentists and practice staff should be provided with:

- good consulting/surgery facilities
- space for sterilisation and preparation of instruments
- materials and equipment storage.

Staff Representatives and Safety Committees – it's the law . . .

By law, trade unions recognised by employers can appoint safety representatives and, if two or more safety representatives ask for a safety committee, the employer must set one up. Union appointed safety representatives have a right to inspect the workplace, to

 Make a Note

The Health and Safety Executive believes that similar arrangements for safety representatives and safety committees can be advantageous even if not required by law.

investigate accidents and complaints from staff about health and safety and to make representations to employers on health and safety matters. Most practices will not have safety representatives and safety committees, though some do.

   Since both employers and employees have health and safety duties, employers will find it helpful if employees contribute to the development and improvement of health and safety procedures. If a safety committee is not practicable, dentists can consider other ways of involving and consulting their staff.

 Make a Note

Dentists may nominate a member of staff to serve as a safety officer and monitor standards. The practice manager could undertake this duty. The safety officer should report to the practice owner as the employer cum-controller of the premises.

PREMISES CHECKLIST

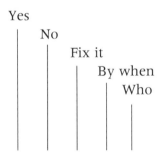

Yes
| No
  | Fix it
    | By when
      | Who

- Is the building maintained in a safe condition without a risk to health?
- Do the premises comply with applicable building codes and regulations?
- Is there a safe means of entrance and exit for staff?
- Are there designated and clearly marked fire exits?
- Do the dentists understand who has the responsibility for maintaining the building?
- Is adequate lighting and ventilation provided in all areas?

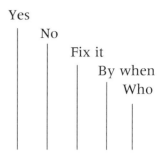

Yes
No
Fix it
By when
Who

- Is there disabled access to the premises?
- Are there adequate toilet facilities?
- Is a non-smoking policy in place and enforced?
- Are there adequate rest and changing areas for staff?
- Is adequate, comfortable seating available?
- Is the reception/waiting area visible to the receptionist?
- Do reception and examination areas assure patients of privacy during interviews, examinations and treatment?

DUTIES TO OTHER USERS OF PRACTICE PREMISES

Although the primary purpose of the Health and Safety at Work Act 1974 is to ensure the safety of employees it also applies to all persons who enter the premises – staff employed by a health authority working on the premises, visitors, patients and tradesmen such as postmen, window cleaners, builders and electricians. Even your mother-in-law . . .

The law requires dentists to conduct their practices in such a way as to ensure, as far as is reasonably practicable, that all persons not in their employment who could be affected are not exposed to risks to their health and safety.

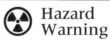 **Hazard Warning**

The Act imposes a duty on the dentist as the 'controller' of the premises to ensure the safety of anyone who legitimately visits the premises.

A health authority or a private landlord may also have a duty under the licence or lease, and may also be liable if an accident occurs.

This is very dull stuff but it is important.

This part of the Act links up with the civil liability of an occupier of premises under the Occupier's Liability Act of 1957. It may be assumed that the standards expected under the Act are equal to the 'duty of care' under the Occupier's Liability Act owed to all persons legitimately entering the premises.

Under the civil law it is advisable for a dentist to anticipate who might be directly affected and to ensure that the premises are safe. The practice owner would be well advised to consider whether there are any potential hazards for elderly or infirm patients.

The key difference between this duty and that to the dentist's own staff is that the staff should be provided with a *written* safety policy, should be instructed and supervised on safety matters and specific arrangements should be made for their health, safety and welfare.

EMPLOYER'S LIABILITY

Don't give up yet – we're on the home run!

The Employer's Liability (EL) (Compulsory Insurance) Act 1969 requires an employer to have adequate insurance and to display a certificate to that effect. New regulations on 1 January 1999 introduced some new requirements for EL cover in the UK. The new regulations supplement the 1969 regulations which remain in force.

Want to know what they are – of course you do!

The latest legislation has increased the minimum level of insurance cover required by employers to £5 million and employers will be required to keep certificates of insurance for 40 years. Yes, and you thought dental records had to be kept for a long time!

Other legislation details the duties of the occupier of premises to ensure safety.

 Make a Note

Although key responsibilities lie with the practice owner, some duties lie with the staff. Employers and employees should co-operate to provide a safe place of work. Employees should take reasonable care of their own health and safety and that of others who may be affected by their errors and omissions. They should co-operate with their employer or any other person – such as a health and safety inspector – who has responsibilities under the Act.

Practice premises must also be covered by adequate public liability insurance and a certificate to that effect must be displayed. The Occupier's Liability Acts 1957 and 1984 regulates the duty which an occupier of premises owes to his or her visitors in respect of damages due to the state of the premises or to things which have been done or which have not been done on them. Generally this means premises must have adequate lighting, safe stairways and all that good common sense stuff.

HERE'S THE STUFF THE STAFF ARE RESPONSIBLE FOR

- Employees have a responsibility for health and safety with regard to themselves, their colleagues and their patients.
- To abide by health and safety rules of the practice.
- To report anything which could compromise health and safety to the person in charge.

Every employee (and indeed any other person) is under a duty not to interfere intentionally or recklessly with, or misuse anything provided for the purposes of health, safety and welfare. This protects appliances and arrangements to ensure people's safety, such as fire escapes, fire extinguishers and hazard warning notices. This could be extended to include interference with anything provided for welfare purposes, such as cloakroom and refreshment facilities.

ENFORCEMENT

The Act covers all places of employment and the HSE therefore has the right to inspect dental practices. The HSE has divided the country into areas, and each has its own team of inspectors. One group of inspectors is responsible for the 'health services', which includes dental practice premises.

 Make a Note

Inspectors normally give notice of their visits and ring to make an appointment. Occasionally, however, a visit may be 'reactive' in response to a complaint from an employee or a patient. Sometimes inspectors make an unannounced call simply because it conveniently fits a visit schedule for other premises.

POWERS OF THE INSPECTORS

Inspectors have a warrant of appointment that states their extensive powers, and the dentist may ask to see this for identification. Inspectors have the right to enter any work premises to enforce the Act. They do not have to seek the practice owner's or any other person's permission, neither do they have to give notice of their visits. They may, however, only enter at a 'reasonable time'.

During an investigation the inspector can interview and take written statements from anyone who may have relevant information *(and this could include patients as well as members of the practice staff)*.

The inspector may want to obtain information or establish the facts about an accident or for evidence in legal proceedings. Any information provided will normally be treated as confidential. The information, however, may be subsequently disclosed if a prosecution is brought against the employer.

WHAT ARE THE INSPECTORS LOOKING FOR?

Inspectors will wish to ensure that dentists with more than five staff have a statement of general policy on health and safety and instructions on safety procedures. Since 1 January 1993 they will also be looking for compliance with the requirement to carry out a risk assessment under the Management of Health and Safety at Work Regulations 1999.

Increasingly inspectors are looking for evidence of a good general approach to the management of health and safety but among specific requirements they will seek are:

- A record for accidents.
- Electrical equipment which is in safe working order and properly maintained.
- The normal standards applying to toilet and washing facilities in offices and shops should be met in the practice premises.
- A supply of hot and cold running water. Inspectors may also recommend that wrist operated taps should be fitted in rooms used for examinations and treatment of patients.
- Inspectors will also be concerned about the conditions of the heating plant, the arrangements for storage of drugs, the condition of sterilisers,

standards of heating and lighting and the procedure for the disposal of clinical waste.

IMPROVEMENT AND PROHIBITION NOTICES

After completing the inspection, the inspector will usually approach the person in administrative charge of the premises (often the practice manager) about any improvements to safety procedures and standards that may be required. If these are minor, the inspector will simply ask for them to be put right. If there is something more serious they may write formally, or serve a written notice requiring matters to be remedied. This is called an *improvement notice*. It will specify a time limit of not less than 21 days within which the improvement must be made. **The inspector must inform staff as well as the practice owner of the service of the notice.** A prosecution alleging a specific breach of a statutory provision may also be brought.

If there is a serious risk to health and safety, an inspector may issue a *prohibition notice* forbidding the offending work activity. If the position is very grave, the notice will take immediate effect and work must stop at once. Otherwise a deferred prohibition notice may be issued stopping the work after a specified time.

The improvement and prohibition notices are both served on a person carrying out, or in control of, the work in question. The notice is normally served on the practice owner, unless control of the practice has been delegated to a practice manager.

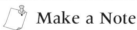 **Make a Note**

The inspector should also advise of the procedure for appeal against the provisions of the notice – very comforting!

A person on whom notice is served may appeal to an employment tribunal within 21 days of the notice being served. An improvement notice is suspended pending the outcome but a prohibition notice remains in force until the appeal is determined. When complied with, notices cease.

Don't mess with the inspectors – they can:

*   issue an improvement notice which specifies the legal requirements being broken, what action is required to put matters right and the period of time allowed

- issue a prohibition notice if there is a risk of serious personal injury
- seize, render harmless or destroy any substance or article considered to be the cause of imminent danger or serious personal injury
- prosecute any person contravening a relevant statutory provision, either instead of or in addition to serving a notice. Summary conviction can result in a fine of up to £20 000 for some offences. Trial on indictment is by a jury and for certain offences (e.g. failure to comply with a prohibition notice) the penalty is imprisonment for up to two years.

The seeds of insomnia – just so you know what you're getting into, here are the Offences and Penalties.

Because the Health and Safety at Work Act is a criminal statute, contravention of its provisions may lead to a fine or imprisonment. Both the employer and his or her staff (as well as any other person on the premises) may be liable to prosecution. Furthermore, failure to carry out any duty under the Act is an offence and could also lead to prosecution. The HSE, as the enforcing authority, has the discretion to decide whether or not to prosecute and this decision is taken after advice from the inspector.

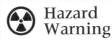 **Hazard Warning**

It is an offence to obstruct an inspector in the performance of duties and to contravene an improvement or prohibition notice.

Not that you would!

Alongside a criminal prosecution of an employer, an employee could sue the employer for damages on the basis of employers' liability law, or simply for negligence. In most prosecutions by the HSE, account will be taken of what was reasonably practicable in the circumstances.

HEALTH AUTHORITY OWNED HEALTH CENTRES

Although a health authority is a Crown Body, it no longer enjoys exemption from prosecution under the Act. Changes in health and safety legislation introduced in 1987 removed crown indemnity from NHS premises.

What could happen?

- Prosecution under criminal law, e.g. fine or imprisonment.
- The employee could sue on the basis of employer's liability law.

- Any visitor could sue under occupier's liability law or the law of negligence.

FIRST AID AND COLLAPSE ROUTINE

No, this is not about reviving you after all this health and safety stuff!

Under the Health and Safety (First Aid) Regulations 1981, all employers must make adequate first aid provisions. Ideally a first aid person should be nominated and all employees should know where the first aid box is kept.

Under GDC guidelines a dentist must ensure that all members of the team are properly trained in cardio-pulmonary resuscitation and prepared to deal with any emergency. Training should include preparing for medical emergencies and practice of resuscitation routines in a simulated emergency. Yearly training can usually be arranged through a local health authority with a certificate of training provided.

Dentists should comply with current guidelines as to the required emergency drugs.

A dentist's emergency equipment and drugs will be checked at a practice inspection.

 Make a Note

There is no obligation to have trained first aiders in a dental practice setting where staff are normally close to hand.

However, there should be a nominal appointed person to take charge of any accident, for example to ensure that an ambulance is called, if necessary, and that the accident is reported.

 Make a Note

Information can also be obtained from the Resuscitation Councils 1997 ABC guidelines on resuscitation and the Dental Practitioners Formulary.

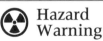 **Hazard Warning**

Failure to comply with guidelines on emergency kit requirements may result in disciplinary action.

A first aid box should be provided.
  It should contain:

Check!

- a guidance card on resuscitation
- individually wrapped sterile adhesive dressings (various sizes)
- individually wrapped triangular bandages
- medium sized individually wrapped sterile unmedicated wound dressings (approximately 10 × 10 cm)
- large sterile individually wrapped unmedicated wound dressings
- other wound dressings
- safety pins
- sterile eye pads and attachments.

 Make a Note

First aid boxes should not contain medication of any kind.

FIRE SAFETY

This is getting serious. Isn't it? Not really, just common sense.

  The Fire Precautions (Workplace) Regulations 1997 require the employer to assess what fire precautions are needed by carrying out a fire risk assessment under the Management of Health and Safety at Work Regulations 1999.

  Employers are required to ensure that proper consideration has been given to fire prevention. The regulations require an employer to ensure that:

- emergency routes and exits are kept clear of obstructions
- they should lead directly to a place of safety
- they should be clearly indicated
- fire detection devices and

 Make a Note

In buildings with more than 20 employees or more than ten working on floors other than the ground floor, the owner of the premises is required to obtain a certificate from the local fire authority regulating the means of escape and marking fire exits.

fire-fighting equipment should be in good working order and regularly checked
- a system should be in place ensuring that, in the event of a fire, the number of people in the practice at that time can be identified.

Premises should be equipped with properly maintained alarms and the employees should be familiar with the means of escape and the routine to be followed in the event of fire. There should be emergency lighting as necessary. Local fire inspectors will ensure that these requirements are complied with.

By the way, make sure that . . .

- a fire can be detected in reasonable time and people warned
- automatic fire detection is considered
- people in the building can get out safely
- there is adequate fire fighting equipment available
- a fire extinguisher is provided for each 200 square metres of floor space with a minimum of one per floor
- all employees know what to do in the event of fire
- fire equipment is checked and maintained.

Emergency routes and exits should:

- be kept free from obstruction at all times
- lead directly to a place of safety
- be appropriately and clearly indicated
- have emergency lighting if required
- open in the direction of escape and in an easy and immediate action.

   See, told you – common sense. Now check out the checklist . . .

FIRE CHECKLIST

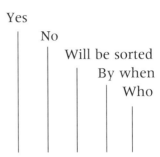

Yes

No

Will be sorted

By when

Who

- Does the practice ensure that all appropriate fire-fighting equipment is available?
- Is fire-fighting equipment serviced regularly?
- Are escape routes and exits appropriately signed?
- Are all fire exits kept clear?
- Are extinguishers appropriately signed?
- Are fire alarms and smoke alarms installed and regularly maintained and tested?
- Are practice staff trained in responses if a fire is detected?
- Is a fire drill practised regularly?
- Is a fire drill notice displayed in the practice?
- Do staff have written protocols about fire procedures?

ELECTRICITY REGULATIONS

You look like a bright spark – sort this lot out!

Did you know, a dentist's responsibilities concerning the supply and use of electricity come under the Electricity at Work Regulations 1989. Well you do now! The regulations are concerned with the safety of both the fixed supply to the premises and any moveable (portable) appliances.

 Make a Note

In the event of someone having a 'shocking time', or worse, if you can show evidence of regular inspection and testing this would be fundamental to the defence that all reasonable steps had been taken to comply with the requirements of the legislation.

Electrical equipment must be in good working order at all times and all earthed equipment and most leads and plugs connected to equipment should have an occasional combined inspection and test by an appropriately trained person to identify any faults which may not be found by a visual check. The HSE has suggested intervals of up to five years in low risk environments depending on the type of equipment used.

Electrical equipment should be checked regularly.

• There should be regular visual inspections of all electrical appliances, including the connection to the mains plug.
• It should be regularly tested by a qualified electrician.
• Records should be kept of all inspections and tests.

There are contract electricians who will provide this type of service. They put little stickers on things to show they've tested them. They'll even remember when they last checked you out and come around and do you again – when the time (and the price) is right.

Before you make the next of tea or coffee, give some thought to the electric kettle – is it safe?

ELECTRICITY CHECKLIST

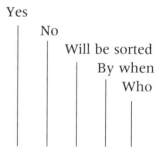

	Yes	No	Will be sorted	By when	Who
• Have you got a programme for ensuring that electrical equipment is safe at all times?					
• Is electrical equipment installed by appropriate contractors?					
• Is all electrical equipment earthed?					
• Is all electrical equipment provided with fuses of the correct amperage?					

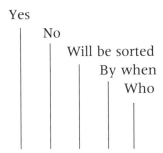

- Is all electrical equipment maintained regularly and a record kept?
- Is electrical wiring checked regularly to inspect for cable or plug damage?
- Are staff vigilant for the possibility of equipment overheating – who should they tell?

COSHH REGULATIONS

These sound like a left over from a communist regime. They're not. They're much worse than that!

The Control of Substances Hazardous to Health Regulations 1999 (COSHH) set out a legal framework for the management of health risks from exposure to hazardous substances used at work. They aim to prevent occupational ill health by encouraging employers to assess and prevent or control risks from exposure to hazardous substances in a systematic and practical way.

 Make a Note

The regulations apply to most hazardous substances except those covered by their own legislation, such as asbestos, lead and material producing ionising radiations.

The regulations set out the measures that employers and employees have to take. Failure to comply exposes people to risk and constitutes an offence under the HSW Act. Hazardous substances include those labelled as dangerous (toxic, harmful, irritant or corrosive).

The most likely substances that a dentist might have to worry about include:

- materials used in dental practice
- certain cleaning fluids

- phenolics
- formaldehyde and glutaraldehyde used as chemical disinfectants
- clinical waste and pathological specimens containing pathogenic organisms.

 Make a Note

All suppliers of materials are required to provide material data sheets which will define the likely hazard.

Risks to health from substances administered in the course of medical treatment, including examination, treatment or administration for the purpose of research are excluded from the provisions.

All employers need to consider how COSHH applies to their employees and working environment. For most dentists compliance should be simple and straightforward.

Here's what you do:

- get hazardous substances identified
- assess the risk to health and what precautions are required
- record precautions in writing
- introduce measures to prevent or control exposure
- ensure that control measures are used, equipment is properly maintained and procedures observed
- inform and instruct employees about the risks and precautions to be taken.

In applying the COSHH regulations, the following risk management assessment should be applied:

- identify each hazardous substance
- assess the risk to those who might contact it
- prevent or control the risk
- inform, train and supervise staff appropriately
- record the assessment.

GOOD MERCURY HYGIENE

An assessment of the risks posed by mercury is required under the COSHH regulations above. Dentists and staff who are regularly exposed to mercury and its vapour should undergo regular monitoring to ensure that their exposure falls within the recommended limits.

Mercury checklist:

- ensure good surgery ventilation
- use a funnel when filling the mercury reservoir to prevent spillage
- place the amalgamator in a shallow tray lined with aluminium foil to catch any droplets
- have a mercury spillage kit available and ensure that staff know of procedures to follow if a spill occurs
- ensure that all staff receive regular biological monitoring which can often be arranged with local health authority occupational health departments.

 Hazard Warning

All staff involved in the handling of mercury should be aware of the potential hazards it poses and be trained in the safe handling procedures to deal with its accidental spillage.

 Make a Note

The overall risks of mercury can be greatly reduced if encapsulated amalgam is used.

WASTE DISPOSAL

Just like going to the bottle bank – well nearly!

The Environmental Protection Act 1990 places a duty of care on dentists to sort their waste, store it safely in a suitable container and arrange for its safe disposal.

Detailed record keeping and documentation is required to track disposal routes (Environmental Protection (Duty of Care) Regulations 1991). Dental practitioners should have a practice policy for the safe collection and disposal of waste.

Waste must be segregated into clinical, non-clinical, special waste and sharps.

 Make a Note

Waste disposal basic requirements:

- Have a written practice waste disposal policy.
- Arrange for safe transportation and collection of waste and subsequent safe disposal in accordance with current legislation.
- If in doubt regard any waste as clinical.

Prescription Only Medicines, waste amalgam and unspent LA cartridges must be treated as special waste.

> **⚛ Hazard Warning**
>
> Mixing clinical and non-clinical waste automatically classifies it as clinical, which is more expensive to dispose of.

Non-clinical waste is material such as paper, plastic etc, whereas clinical waste is that contaminated by blood, saliva, or other body fluids. If in doubt it may be advisable to classify the waste as clinical and dispose of it accordingly.

Clinical waste may still be transported in yellow UN approved clinical waste sacks until 31 December 2001. However from 1 January 2002 it will have to be transported in UN approved rigid containers (Carriage of Dangerous Goods (Classification, Packaging and Labelling) and Use of Transportable Pressure Receptacles Regulations 1996). Sharps must be sealed in UN type approved 'sharps' containers to BS7320. So now you know!

Clinical waste and sharps must only be collected by authorised persons and documentation of the waste content must be provided and records of the transfer held by both parties.

Transfer notes may cover repeated transfers up to one year. You are required to hang on to documentation for a period of two years.

The Special Waste Regulations 1996 apply to prescribed medicines and other waste classified as irritant, harmful, toxic, carcinogenic or corrosive. Partially discharged local anaesthetic cartridges must be disposed of as special waste. If these are disposed of via the sharps box, then the container

> ☕ . . . for a thrilling, bodice ripping read, here's the relevant legislation. Great to read at bedtime – if it doesn't send you to sleep, nothing will!
>
> • Environmental Protection Act 1990.
> • Environmental Protection (Duty of Care) Regulations 1991.
> • Special Waste Regulations 1996 as amended.
> • Carriage of Dangerous Goods (Classification, Packaging and Labelling) and Use of Transportable Pressure Receptacles Regulations 1996.

must be disposed of as special waste. Fully discharged cartridges are not regarded as special waste.

Consignment notices must be used at each stage of the disposal of special waste and kept for three years. Waste amalgam and mercury are regarded as controlled waste and must not be sent through the post. An authorised person must collect them and a transfer note should be completed.

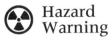

Hazard Warning

Dentists who fail to dispose of waste appropriately face prosecution. The safe disposal of waste is also a requirement of the GDC (Maintaining Standards Para 6.4).

WASTE DISPOSAL CHECKLIST

Important stuff this, go through the checklist carefully. It might be a job for the practice manager but at the end of the day, the dentist is the boss and will be the one to get their neck in a sling if something's not right.

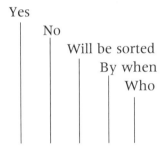

- Are you aware of the different types of waste and the requirements for the correct disposal of each?
- Is the practice waste correctly categorised, stored and disposed of?
- Is clinical waste stored in yellow sacks?
- Are all staff members trained in its disposal?
- Do staff only handle clinical waste when using heavy duty rubber gloves?
- Are clinical waste sacks disposed of when they are two-thirds full?
- Are systems in place for the correct transfer of waste?
- Is waste collected by an authorised person?
- Has the practice checked the certificate of registration of the waste remover?
- When clinical waste is removed is a signature obtained by the practice?
- Are transfer notes kept for two years?

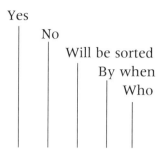

```
Yes
 │ No
 │  │ Will be sorted
 │  │  │ By when
 │  │  │  │ Who
 │  │  │  │  │
 │  │  │  │  │
```

- Are sharps sealed in UN type approved 'sharps' containers?
- Does the practice realise that medicines and partially discharged local anaesthetic cartridges are classified as special waste?
- Are consignment notes for special waste kept for three years?

PRESSURE SYSTEMS REGULATIONS

Under the Provision and Use of Work Equipment Regulations 1998 employers must ensure that all work equipment is safe.

All staff that use autoclaves within the practice should be trained to use them according to the manufacturer's instructions. Periodic checks must be carried out in accordance with a written scheme drawn up by a competent person who should be a qualified engineer.

Get your head around this and be safe:

- The design of compressors and autoclaves should meet relevant British standards.
- The autoclave should have a safety valve, a reducing valve, an isolating or stop valve, a pressure indicator and a drainage system.
- The maximum allowable working pressure should be clearly marked on the autoclave.

 More information for the really sad . . .

Pressure systems, which will include compressors and autoclaves, are governed by the Pressure Equipment Regulations 1999 and the Pressure Systems Safety Regulations 2000, which came into force on 21 February 2000. The latter regulations re-enact with amendments, the Pressure Systems and Transportable Gas Containers Regulations 1989 and revoke regulation 21(6) of and Schedule 6 to the CDGCPL Regulations and Regulation 3 of and Schedule 2 to the Carriage of Dangerous Goods (Amendment) Regulations 1999.

Here's what the regulations call for:

- A written scheme of examination drawn up by a competent person.
- Periodic examinations are carried out and recorded.
- Regular service and maintenance is carried out according to manufacturer's instructions and each autoclave has a written service schedule.
- A programme of staff training in the use of autoclaves.
- Equipment requiring regular service is labelled to identify next service date.

PRESSURE SYSTEM CHECKLIST

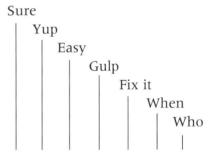

Sure
Yup
Easy
Gulp
Fix it
When
Who

- Are risks from pressure systems minimised in the practice?
- Have all staff been trained in the use of the equipment?
- Does each piece of equipment have clear operating instructions?
- Is there a written schedule for periodic inspection and testing of all pressure system equipment?
- Does the scheme cover all protective devices, pressure vessels and pipelines?
- Are the inspections carried out by someone who is competent to do so?
- Are staff trained in emergency procedures in respect of pressure systems?
- Does the practice have pressure vessel insurance to provide cover in the event of damage to a pressure vessel?

COMPUTERS

How do you know you're in a dental surgery? Look at the PC, there'll be Tippex on the screen!

If computers are used in a practice (is there a practice left that doesn't use computers?) there are responsibilities in two areas:

1   For regular VDU users there are responsibilities under the Health and Safety (Display Screen Equipment) Regulations 1992, to assess the workplace and to take steps to reduce any identified risks. Employees should be trained to use their workstation correctly in order to avoid health problems. The type of training and the date provided should be recorded.

2   Responsibilities under data protection and other legislation regarding the rights of patients concerning confidentiality and access to clinical records.

 Make a Note

- Analyse workstations and assess and reduce risks.
- Ensure workstations meet minimum requirements.
- Plan work so there are breaks or changes of activity.
- On request arrange eye tests and provide spectacles if special ones are needed.
- Provide health and safety training.

. . . and, register with the Data Protection Registrar if holding patient records on computer.

Data protection legislation protects the individual against potential misuse of personal information held by a data user, e.g. unauthorised disclosure of or inaccurate data and gives the right of access to data of which they are the subject. It has considerable implications for healthcare professionals who maintain computerised and written patient records.

A dentist must register as a data user with the Data Protection Commissioner and comply with a series of data protection principles in a manner that is set out in the Data Protection Act. Registration describes the type of data held and sources and persons to whom data is disclosed. Data must be accurate, up to date, used only for specified and lawful purposes and not disclosed in any way that is incompatible with these purposes.

COMPUTER CHECKLIST

Eeer, shouldn't this be done on a spreadsheet on a computer? Funny how we still buy books! (*Thank goodness – Ed*).

 This is a long list so pay attention. Make a coffee and plough through it.

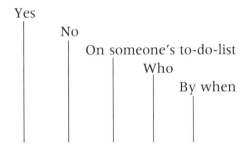

Yes

No

On someone's to-do-list

Who

By when

- Have regular users of DSE (Display Screen Equipment) been identified?
- Do 'computer users' include those people continuously at a screen for longer than one hour at a time, using a PC every day or needing to use a PC to do the job?
- Have the workstations been assessed?
- Have the workstations been upgraded or changed to rectify any problems with the workstation set-up identified at risk assessment?
- Are free eyesight tests regularly offered to all DSE users?
- Are employees aware that they should report any discomfort in working with DSE to their manager?
- Are the computer users instructed and trained in their use?
- Are records kept of workstation assessments, eyesight tests and results, and are corrective appliances offered and details of information and training provided?

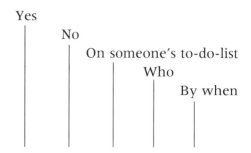

Yes

No

On someone's to-do-list

Who

By when

Equipment:

- Do images on screen flicker or jump?
- Can the user adjust the brightness and contrast controls on the PC? Is instruction required to enable them to do this?
- Can the user tilt or swivel the screen to avoid glare and allow the maintenance of a comfortable posture?
- Is the screen clean and are cleaning materials available?
- Is the keyboard tiltable and separate from the screen (apart from wire connections) allowing the user to adjust the keyboard to suit their needs?
- Does the keyboard have a matt surface to avoid reflective glare?
- Is there sufficient space in front of the keyboard to allow users to rest their wrists whilst keying in or resting?
- Is a wrist rest required and, if so, has it been supplied?
- Is a mouse necessary and has a mouse mat been supplied?
- Is the work area provided adequate to accommodate the range of tasks performed?
- Can unessential items be relocated?
- Is a document holder required and has one been provided?

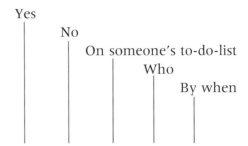

Yes

No

On someone's to-do-list

Who

By when

- Does the work chair allow the user to obtain a comfortable posture and is the seat adjustable for height, lumbar support and tilt?
- Does the user require a footrest (do the feet reach the floor when sitting) and if so has one been provided?

Environment:

- Do the user's legs fit comfortably under the work surface?
- Does the workstation allow a comfortable posture for the user?
- Is lighting appropriate for the tasks being undertaken?
- Is there glare or reflection from the screen and, if so, have steps been taken to control it using window blinds, lighting adjustment or, if the only solution, an antiglare screen?
- Is noise a problem and, if so, what is proposed for its reduction?
- Are temperature and humidity levels appropriate?

Task design and software:

- Is the task designed to ensure variety, allowing the user to take regular breaks to undertake other tasks?

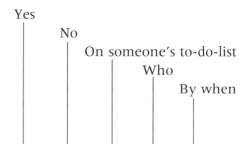

Yes
No
On someone's to-do-list
Who
By when

- Can users take breaks from the
  screen at their own discretion?
- Are users involved in the
  planning, design and
  implementation of tasks?
- Does the software used enable
  users to complete tasks efficiently,
  without presenting unnecessary
  problems or stress?
- Are users fully trained to operate
  the software used and have any
  further training requirements been
  identified?
- Does the software provide on-line
  help and feedback to the user
  (e.g. as error messages, etc.)?
- Is there a system of task checking
  (whereby managers can check the
  amount of work being generated by
  employees) and are employees
  aware of this?

MANUAL HANDLING

This section is not about lifting instruction books or throwing patients out of
the surgery . . .

These regulations place responsibilities on both the employer and
employee to ensure that handling is reduced to a minimum and mechanical
aids are used wherever possible. Training in handling should be given to
all staff and employees must use equipment where it is provided. The
employer must assess the risks taking into account the loads involved, the

environment in which the handling takes place and the individual capacity for carrying out the task.

For the really sad, the legislation is: Manual Handling Operations Regulations 1992 – vintage stuff! Be sure to get a copy, before stocks run out. Be careful lifting it!

MEDICINE STORAGE

Correct medicine storage is essential to ensure that they do not deteriorate. That costs you money and isn't very good for the patients. If you keep any controlled drugs they should be secured in a locked cupboard.

There was a nice little punch up, recently, between a member of staff and her employer. She sued him on the grounds she had been obliged to carry a box of photocopy paper from reception to the paper store. She'd hurt her back and said it was her boss' fault. The case got to the door of the Court and, on advice, settled.

Got a photocopier? You need to know there is at least one stationery company who now deliver copy paper direct to your paper store. Can't tell you which one because that's advertising – but the name sounds like a Nordic invader!

An adequate stock control system should be in place to deal with outdated stocks and ensure minimum stock holding. Strict records should be kept of batch and lot numbers.

Read, learn and inwardly digest the Misuse of Drugs (Safe Custody) Regulations 1973! Try not to go blind . . .

PATHOLOGICAL SPECIMENS

If you decide to use the good old Royal Snail Mail to send patients' specimens to pathology labs for diagnostic opinion or tests you must comply with UN 602 packaging requirements. The outer shipping package must bear the UN packaging specification marking. Only first class letter post, special delivery or data post services must be used. The parcel post must not be used – even though it is cheaper . . .

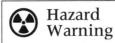

Hazard Warning

Pathological specimens containing Hazard Group 4 pathogens should not be sent through the post.

Any dental practitioner sending a pathological specimen through the post without complying with these requirements may be liable to prosecution, go to jail, pay a huge fine and have their teeth pulled out by a plumber.

I repeat, the dentist should use first class post, special delivery or data post services and should ensure that the pathological specimen is packaged to comply with UN 602 packaging requirements.

The outer package must be labelled

'Packed in compliance with the
Post Office Inland Letter Post
Scheme'

PROTECTIVE CLOTHING

The Personal Protective Equipment at Work Regulations 1992 require an employer to provide protective clothing where it is necessary to ensure safe systems at work.

PPE made or sold in the UK must carry the CE marking and necessary information. Surgery clothing must be of a material that can be washed at a temperature of 65 degrees centigrade – that means hot to you and me. Eye and hand protection should be provided and the employer must ensure that it is used by the employee.

All the stunningly interesting details are to be found in the Personal Protective Equipment at Work Regulations 1992.

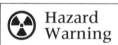 **Hazard Warning**

Gloves

Medical gloves for single use (to BS EN 455) should be worn for relevant clinical procedures. Care should be taken when choosing latex gloves as latex is covered by the COSHH Regulations. So no cutting corners with cheap gloves, no matter how persuasive the rep' may be.

Further advice is contained in the Medical Devices Agency's publication *Latex Sensitisation in the Health Care Setting (use of latex gloves) (DB 9601).*

REPORTING OF INJURIES, DISEASES AND DANGEROUS OCCURRENCES

Otherwise known by the ludicrous acronym (RIDDOR), to find out why, read on, brave heart . . .

The Reporting of Injuries, Diseases and Dangerous Occurrences Regulations 1995 *(See, RIDDOR! Got it now?)* impose duties on employers to notify the Health and Safety Executive of accidents causing death or major injury in the workplace.

These are relevant to dentists because they impose a statutory obligation on all employers to keep a record of accidents occurring on their premises and to notify the Health and Safety Executive of certain serious accidents. The employer is responsible for reporting any accident, dangerous occurrence or a case of an occupational disease, although in some circumstances responsibility lies with the owner of the premises.

It is a very good idea for dentists to **assume that they are responsible** for notifying the HSE even if they do not carry responsibility for the premises. Any notifiable accident must be directly notified to the local office of the HSE by telephone. It is advisable to keep a written record of the call including the name of the

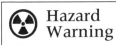 **Hazard Warning**

All accidents must be recorded in a practice accident book, but major accidents must be reported to the Health and Safety Executive immediately by telephone and within ten days on form F2508.

The regulations also require the reporting of certain occupationally related diseases occurring in the workplace.

civil servant receiving it and the details of the accident, occurrence or disease. A written report should be sent to the HSE within ten days.

Notifiable dangerous occurrences are also defined in the Regulations and include explosion, electrical short circuit or overload attended by fire or explosion which resulted in the stoppage of the plant for more than 24 hours. Accidents involving explosion of the compressor or autoclave could therefore be notifiable under these Regulations, as could serious mercury spillage.

Employers must make and keep a record of all reported injuries and dangerous occurrences. Under the Regulations cases of certain diseases must also be reported when a person is carrying out a particular type of work, and in relation to dentistry these include poisoning, TB, hepatitis, anthrax, certain skin diseases and bone cancer arising from radiation.

Make a Note

What do you report? Here's a list of the basics.

• Record any accidents in a practice accident book.
• If a major accident occurs in the practice the HSE must be notified immediately by telephone and within ten days on form F2508.
• Dangerous occurrences must be reported, i.e. if something happens which does not result in an injury but could have done so.
• If an accident happens to an employee in your practice and causes that employee to be absent for three days or more, the HSE must be notified.
• If an employee suffers from a reportable work related disease the HSE must be informed.

If an accident occurs you must record:

• date and time of the accident
• name and occupation of the injured party
• nature of the injury
• where it occurred
• name and address of witnesses and any other relevant information.

WRITTEN RECORDS OF RIDDOR

A record must be kept of all notifiable accidents and dangerous occurrences, so that the employer can monitor these and identify any preventive action that should be taken. Failure to do so could lead to a fine of up to £5000.

GOT THE BUILDERS IN?

 By the way . . .

A dentist need not report an accident to him or herself. See nobody loves you. Not even the Health and Safety Executive!

Serious hazards can arise when building work is in progress. Tea can be spilled and sandwiches dropped in the cement! More seriously, the main contractor, sub-contractor and their employees have the prime duty to carry out their work in a safe manner. Your job, as 'controller' of the premises, is to ensure that your staff, other employees on the premises, patients and visitors are not put at risk. If unavoidable temporary hazards are caused by building operations these should be identified and their risks reduced as far as possible by providing warning notices that can be easily read by everyone using the premises.

When in doubt, ask the local HSE office.

Major incidents which need to be reported include:

Check

• fractures of the skull, spine or pelvis
• fracture of any bone in the arm or leg (except in the wrist, hand, ankle or foot)
• amputation of a hand or foot
• dislocation of the shoulder, hip, knee or spine
• loss of sight in an eye
• loss of consciousness through lack of oxygen
• any other injury resulting in a person injured or being admitted to hospital as an inpatient for more than 24 hours, unless detained only for observation.

Notifiable dangerous occurrences include:

• explosion
• electrical short circuit.

SAFETY SIGNS

For the detailed low-down on all this, try the Health and Safety Executive. In the meantime, here are the basics:

The Health and Safety (Safety Signs and Signals) Regulations 1996 apply to all workplaces and place a duty on employers to use a safety sign wherever a hazard exists that cannot be adequately controlled by any other means.

This means, when everything else has been done to remove the hazard, safety signs should be used to reduce the risk further. Fire safety signs are within the Regulations and include information on emergency exits, escape routes and the identification of fire fighting equipment.

> ### Checklist ✔
> - All safety signs should carry a pictogram.
> - Fire-fighting equipment and unobstructed fire escape routes must be adequately sign-posted and contain information on assembly points.
> - A safety sign must be displayed locating the first aid facilities and identifying the designated person.
>
> You should have a minimum of the following safety signs within the practice:
>
> - *Fire safety signs* – these must provide safety information on escape routes, emergency exits, location of fire fighting equipment and a means of giving warning in the event of a fire.
> - *First aid* – where first aid facilities are located and the designated person.

CROSS INFECTION CONTROL

If you don't know most of this stuff already, you shouldn't be a dentist! So, look upon it as a refresher!

Dentists have a duty to take adequate measures to prevent cross infection and breach of this duty would almost certainly lead to a charge of serious professional misconduct (4.1 GDC's Maintaining Standards 1997).

An allegation of failure to exercise infection control may be brought against a dentist working in the General Dental Services by the health authority, who may refer the matter for disciplinary action.

So, keep out of trouble, make sure all dental staff are adequately trained in the practice procedures and routines which should be in place for sterilisation and cross infection control.

It would be sensible to put in place nationally accepted guidelines on these issues, with the use of disposable items as often as possible and effective cleaning and disinfection of surfaces.

Each practice should have an infection control policy. Precautions should be consistently applied to all patients. The practice cross infection control policy should be clear and concise and each member of staff should be adequately trained in its application.

 Make a Note

You need a policy to cover this – it's important stuff. The basics are:

- adopt universal cross infection control procedures
- all staff must be adequately trained
- infection control policy displayed in each surgery
- universal infection control procedures used at all times.

GENERAL CONSIDERATIONS

. . . and other well-known military leaders!

All dental staff involved in clinical procedures must be vaccinated against Hepatitis B with booster doses given five years after completion of the primary course.

Surgery clothing, which should be provided by employers, should be washed at a temperature of 65 degrees centigrade, to eliminate any potential microbial contamination.

Hand and eye protection is vital for clinical staff with good quality non-sterile medical gloves being worn for clinical procedures and changed after each use. The dentist should ensure that gloves used are fit for their purpose. Masks should also be worn and changed after every patient.

 Make a Note

It is also advisable that staff have immunity to other common illnesses such as diphtheria, whooping cough, polio, rubella, tetanus, and TB.

CJD AND RISK OF TRANSMISSION DURING DENTAL TREATMENT

. . . or the mad cow section.

Transmissible spongiform encephalopathies (TSEs) are fatal degenerative prion disorders of humans and animals. There are several recognised TSEs including BSE in cattle, scrapie in sheep and Creutzfeldt-Jacob disease in humans.

 Make a Note

To identify patients in these at risk groups, medical history forms should be amended to include the question:

'Did you, as a child or since, have brain surgery, growth hormone treatment before the mid 1980s or have a close relative with CJD?'

The TSEs are caused by abnormal prions (proteinaceous infectious particles). In humans the TSEs are inherited, acquired or sporadic.

The acquired human prion diseases include sporadic, iatrogenic and variant CJD (vCJD). Variant CJD is rare and is geographically located in Europe.

The BDA produced a revised cross infection control booklet in January 2000, which advised dentists that those known or suspected to be infected and those at risk require special infection control procedures.

At risk groups are:

- recipients of hormone derived from human pituitary glands, e.g. growth hormone or gonadotrophin
- recipients of human dura mater grafts
- persons with a family history of CJD.

It is essential to distinguish between those who are known or suspected to have CJD and those who are potentially at risk of developing it.

Be sure to go through this list and get it right.

Check

- All equipment used in patients with known CJD must be destroyed after use, hence single-use equipment should be used.
- In patients at risk of CJD, current guidance is that if the procedure involves brain, spinal cord or eye tissue, the instruments must be destroyed after use. If these tissues are not involved, the instruments can be re-used, BUT they must be sterilised under very stringent conditions.
- If a patient has CJD the dental handpiece must be disposed of after use. In those at risk the handpiece and other instruments can be autoclaved in a non-porous load steam steriliser 134–137 degrees centigrade for a single cycle of 18 minutes or six successive cycles of three minutes each, although this is not believed to be completely effective. Dental handpieces must not be attached to the waterline of the dental unit.

Be sure you take a good medical history and, just to be helpful, the Department of Health advises you to follow universal cross infection control procedures.

This includes scrubbing all instruments prior to autoclaving. There is no evidence of transmission of vCJD in the literature and the risk is currently the same as with any other surgical procedure.

 Make a Note

Future research by SEAC will examine whether the prion proteins involved are present in the dental pulp and other oral sites.

Dento-legal advice is to comply with Department of Health and BDA guidance. The Scottish Executive Health Department is also currently examining the issue and may produce specific guidance in the near future.

INFECTED CLINICIAN?

Believe you may have been infected with HIV, hepatitis viruses or other blood borne viruses? You have an ethical responsibility to obtain medical advice, including any necessary testing. If you are found to be

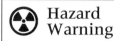

Hazard Warning

Make sure you maintain patient confidentiality at all times. That includes making sure staff don't gossip!

infected, you must seek appropriate medical supervision. Counselling is available for you, particularly in relation to clinical practice. Changes to your clinical practice may be required which may include ceasing to practice or the exclusion of exposure-prone procedures.

WATER LINES

Water and airlines should be fitted with anti-retraction valves to prevent back contamination of water supplies. It is also advised that handpieces are run through with water for 20–30 seconds after the treatment of each patient and at the start of the day for two minutes.

 Make a Note

Most modern dental surgery equipment will comply with these regulations. If in doubt check it out with the manufacturer.

The Water Supply (Water Fittings) Regulations 1999 protect against back-flow to the mains water supply. Dentists must add an air gap to the water supply to the surgery.

DISINFECTION OF HANDPIECES AND IMPRESSIONS

The Medical Devices Regulations 1994 require that handpieces and other equipment should be sterilised prior to being sent for repair. Dental impressions should be adequately disinfected prior to sending to the lab. Disinfect in accordance with the instructions of the manufacturer of the material used. Dental labs should be informed that disinfection has taken place.

Infection control policy should cover the following issues:

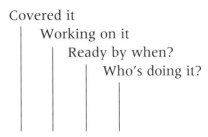

Covered it
   Working on it
      Ready by when?
         Who's doing it?

- Immunisation of staff.
- Use of protective clothing, gloves, masks etc.
- Personal hygiene.
- Cleaning and sterilisation of instruments, equipment and work areas.
- Use and disposal of sharps.
- Clinical waste disposal procedures.
- Procedures for dealing with injuries and accidents involving potentially infectious material.
- Confidentiality of patient information.
- Staff training.
- The prohibition of eating, drinking and smoking except in designated areas.
- The use and maintenance of decontamination equipment, e.g. how to load and operate autoclaves, disinfectors and hot air ovens.
- Handling of toxic materials.
- Correct disposal of different types of waste.
- Disinfection of impressions and sterilisation of handpieces.

INFECTION CONTROL CHECKLIST

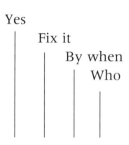

Yes
Fix it
By when
Who

- Does the dentist ensure that all equipment has been sterilised or adequately disinfected?
- Does the dentist put disposable coverings in place where necessary?
- Does the dentist treat all patients as potentially infectious?
- Does the dentist wear gloves, protective clothing and eyewear if required?
- Does the dentist handle sharps carefully and only re-sheath using a device?
- Does the dentist dispose of sharps and segregate waste according to regulations?
- Are infection control policies in place, enforced and include blood borne pathogens and universal precautions?
- Do all staff members receive training on infection control annually? Is this documented in their personnel file?
- Do sterilisation procedures follow manufacturers guidelines/infection control standards of the profession?
- Are sterile supplies dated and checked?
- Does the dentist ensure appropriate medical history taking with particular reference to recent concerns re the transmission of CJD?
- Does the dentist ensure that staff are adequately trained in universal sterilisation and cross infection control procedures?

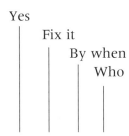

- Does the dentist have a practice infection control policy?
- Does the dentist maintain patient confidentiality in an appropriate manner?
- Does the dentist apply universal infection control procedures?

INOCULATION INJURIES

Inoculation injuries, that means those where a contaminated object or substance breaches the integrity of the skin, must be properly dealt with. The dentist should follow a recommended protocol for their treatment.

Here's what to look for in a protocol:

INJURY

- Make the wound bleed.
- Wash in running water.
- Assess the hepatitis antibody status of the victim.
- Refer to local consultant in communicable diseases.
- Record accident (RIDDOR).

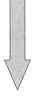

 Make a Note

Every health authority or health board will have at least one designated specialist in communicable diseases based in the Department of Public Health Medicine, who will generally be able to give advice on prophylaxis following inoculation injuries.

CONTACT WITH BLOOD

First rule – all staff should take every precaution to avoid contact with blood.
Second rule – read the first rule!

Blood provides a source or reservoir for any pathogenic organism, a mode of transmission, and if precautions are not taken, there will be a mode of entry into the new host. Much anxiety revolves around the acquisition of HIV but the much greater risk is of acquisition of hepatitis.

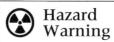 **Hazard Warning**
It is essential that all staff understand the considerable importance of taking care to avoid contact with blood.

Clear protocols should be established to ensure that the risk of contact with blood or any other body fluid is minimised.

Have you got some guidance and rules. No? Try these:

- wash hands between each patient
- use paper towels
- wear gloves and change them after each patient
- gloves should be well fitting and give good sensitivity
- wear a mask, particularly if the procedure is creating an aerosol
- wear protective glasses
- use disposable bibs.

To sterilise instruments:

- soak in soapy water
- transfer to ultrasonic bath
- ensure no residual debris
- hand scrub wearing heavy duty gloves
- autoclave according to manufacturer's directions
- oil, flush out and autoclave handpieces between every appointment and store appropriately
- ensure sufficient handpieces and instruments to permit satisfactory sterilisation procedures.

. . . and, by the way, ensure that there is a written policy for cross infection control.

VENTILATION

This section is a breath of fresh air!

The Workplace (Health, Safety and Welfare) Regulations 1992 require enclosed workplaces to be ventilated with sufficient fresh or purified air.

Basic stuff – makes you wonder what they do all day in the Palace of Westminster – doesn't it?

- Windows must be of reasonable size and able to be opened.
- Any air supply must be from a clean source.
- Sufficient air movement must be available to ensure constant fresh air supply.
- If necessary the requirement for mechanical ventilation should be considered.

 Make a Note

Consideration must be given to adequate ventilation where sedation gases are used for inhalation anaesthesia – see *Anaesthetic Agents: controlling exposure under COSHH*, available from HSE Books.

RADIATION HAZARDS

Dentists must comply with the Ionising Radiations Regulations 1999, which revoke the 1985 regulations of the same name. The Ionising Radiation (Medical Exposure) Regulations 2000 revoke the Ionising Radiation (POPUMET) Regulations 1988. Got that – or do you want to read it again? Might be useful background info for the pub trivia quiz!

You might guess the Ionising Radiation (Medical Exposure) Regulations 2000 place certain duties on employers and practitioners/operators of radiation equipment.

For example:

The employer shall ensure that written protocols are in place for every type of standard radiological practice for each equipment.

 Make a Note

The regulations require that individual medical exposures are justified.

Here's what you've got to do to comply with the regulations and keep out of jail:

- Notify local Health and Safety Executive of radiation usage in the practice.
- Decide if a Radiation Protection Adviser (RPA) is required. Dental practices may be exempt. However the exemption from this covers only the operation of standard dental radiographic units for intra-oral and extra-oral sources.
- Appoint a Radiation Protection Supervisor.
- Ensure that equipment meets required standards of radiation safety.
- Provide Local Rules, which must include the name of the RPS, a description of the controlled area and any special provisions of a local nature.
- A radiation safety assessment must be carried out every three years by a 'competent authority'. This will either be National Radiological Protection Board or a local medical physics department.
- All equipment must meet all standards as recommended in 1994 guidelines and must be serviced and maintained according to manufacturer's specification.
- Personal monitoring for staff by a dosemeter is required if they take more than 150 intra-oral or 50 OPGs each week.
- Staff must be appropriately trained. Dental nurses can be trained to take radiographs, e.g. OPGs.
- Local rules must include a contingency plan to specify what needs to be done following equipment malfunction.

Guidelines produced in 1994 say:

- Techniques using film holders and beam aiming devices should be adopted for bitewing and periapical radiography by 1998, with rectangular collimation adopted for bitewing and periapical radiography by 2001.
- Radiographic equipment with effective operating potentials less than 50kV should be replaced by 2001.

The GDC requires a dentist who owns or operates an X-ray machine to comply

 Make a Note

Lead aprons do not have to be routinely used. However it may be appropriate to display a notice stating why they are not used.

with all regulations and operate safe practice to safeguard patients and members of the dental team and others. Failure to do so may result in a charge of serious professional misconduct. So, watch out!

CARE AND MAINTENANCE OF DENTAL EQUIPMENT AND HANDPIECES

You've spent all this money on your gleaming kit – better try to look after it!

First things first – equipment must be installed by competent persons and, if necessary, there must be formal and recorded maintenance, testing or servicing by competent persons, probably from the manufacturers' engineers or agents.

Where formal arrangements are not necessary, PUWER (one more for the anoraks: The Provision and Use of Work Equipment Regulations 1998) require that all equipment is maintained adequately and in accordance with manufacturers' instructions, that it is fit for the purpose for which it is purchased and that it is used only for that purpose.

Got a bargain at a car-boot sale?

Any equipment purchased secondhand is regarded as new to the purchaser when you start to use it, therefore obtain all records of maintenance, testing or servicing from that nice Mr Trotter.

Anyone using equipment must be trained in its operation, how to switch it off in case of emergency or malfunction and how to deal with an emergency.

 Make a Note

In relation to health and safety, all equipment used in a workplace comes under The Provision and Use of Work Equipment Regulations 1998 (PUWER). These cover not only specifically dental equipment but also general items such as photocopiers.

Specialised equipment may come under other regulations such as The Pressure Systems Safety Regulations 2000 (compressors), The Ionising Radiations Regulations 1999 (X-ray equipment) and The Personal Protective Equipment at Work Regulations 1992 (gloves, eyewear and so on).

Holidaying in Hong Kong and bringing back a nice new whizzo-dubrey, thingamajig?

The Medical Devices Directive requires that instructions for use, in English, accompany new kit and they must be kept on file as soon as the

dental team has become fully conver-
sant with the equipment. Information
about the supplying company together
with the service record, particularly for
autoclaves and X-ray units must be
kept where this is already a mandatory
requirement.

 Make a Note

The representative of the
dental equipment supplier
should generally be expected
to provide instructions about
the use of any significant piece
of equipment to supplement
the written information upon
commissioning of new
equipment.

Make a note of the date of installation. That way you'll know when the
guarantee runs out! Keep a note of
the contact person of the supplier
for technical service and don't bin
service reports and correspondence concerning the equipment. File it. You
never know . . .

All equipment in the surgery should be listed together with serial
number (where appropriate), date of supply, name and address of supplier,
initial purchase price, telephone number for technical support and contact
person. Check that valid instructions for use of the equipment exist and a
contact number for the supplier is available to obtain any missing
information.

Make a note in the diary of the dates for maintenance.

Who, internally, is responsible for looking after the kit? Sort it out and
note it on the file. Make sure that all maintenance procedures are recorded
and kept with the equipment file and that all service reports are stored in the
equipment file.

CLEANING AND MAINTENANCE OF ROTARY HANDPIECES

How come these things cost
sooooo much?

The price of kit is a good topic
for another book *(yes, but not now!
Ed)*. Well, the least we can do is
look after the damned things!
Good maintenance regimes will
ensure maximum life and
breakdowns and repairs will be
minimised.

 Make a Note

Be sure to follow the manufacturers'
instructions regarding the
maintenance of these products and to
use their recommended, proprietary
care sprays. They may vary from
manufacturer to manufacturer.

There is also the minor imperative that you bung these things into the mouths of your punters – so they need to be sparkling, dazzling, eat-your-dinner-off-them, clean.

From an infection control point of view the cleaning of all internal lumina of the handpiece is essential prior to sterilisation, ideally in a vacuum autoclave (as recommended in the British Dental Association Advice Sheet A12 – did you know that?).

Maintenance sprays should include both surfactants, to aid removal of encrusted proteineous deposits, together with vegetable-based lubricant to protect all moving parts within the handpiece.

There are now automatic systems available in addition to the traditional manual use of aerosol cans of care spray. The new whizzo automatic systems ensure the thorough internal and, in some cases, external cleaning and lubrication of dental handpieces. In addition, precise oil dosage eliminates potential waste. To be frank, these systems don't come cheap but they do have the advantage of ensuring the working life of the instrument is prolonged.

There is evidence that, with proper cleaning and maintenance, the frequency of breakdowns can be halved. Some manufacturers have significantly increased their warranty periods as a result. Be sure to follow manufacturers' instructions precisely.

Have you got a practice policy for handpiece maintenance and sterilisation? If not why not? It's not rocket science . . .

The first step is to find out which rotary instruments are being used over at your place. Ask the dental supplier or handpiece manufacturer for the maintenance procedure for each instrument. Then be sure everyone does it.

Write a plain English, dummy's guide, easy to understand for all the practice staff so they know what to do.

Provide a simple, standard procedure for everyone to follow prior to sterilisation. Make it really clear and, if you can, include some pictures of the sequence you want followed.

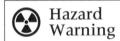 **Hazard Warning**

Chemical wipes should not be used as these can damage both the surface of the instrument and the 0-ring sealants within the instrument.

 Make a Note

Instruments should be lubricated prior to sterilisation and should not be done again after sterilisation, as the handpiece would be re-contaminated and excess oil could affect tooth surfaces prior to adhesive dentistry.

Make sure you always have plenty of stocks of care spray – make running out a hanging offence!

An instrument stand with drip pad should be used to ensure vertical drainage of excess lubricant and condensed water from the instrument. Perhaps a better way is an automatic cleaning/lubrication system. They are more expensive but ensure optimal maintenance. The kit costs loadsa dough, so spend the extra and really look after it. Treat yourself!

What happens when it goes crunch, grind, whirr and dies?

In the event of breakdown, clean the instrument externally **and** internally, then autoclave prior to sending it off to get fixed. Confirmation of sterilisation must be included in the package. Ideally the chosen repairer should work to a defined quality standard (ISO 9000) and be authorised by the manufacturer employing exclusively original spare parts that meet the manufacturer's precise specifications.

 Hazard Warning

It is an offence to send unsterilised medical devices through the post and could lead to prosecution, jail, bankruptcy, divorce, disgrace, dishonour and shame.

SHARP ENOUGH?

Sharpening techniques are important elements of maintenance. New scalers and curettes are delivered with a factory-sharp cutting edge and will remove calculus with the minimum of effort causing the least possible trauma to the surface of the tooth, root or gingival tissue.

Over time the cutting edge will be dulled by contact with the hard tooth enamel and the sterilisation process. Calculus will be burnished if treated with a blunt blade, making removal much harder. This means harder work for the operator and a longer procedure time. And, we all know, time is money. So, be sharp and stay sharp!

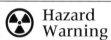 **Make a Note**

It is far better to sharpen the instruments little and often rather than wait for the cutting edges to become dull. Sharpening blunt instruments requires far more time and effort.

Blunt instruments carry another risk – skidding, which may lead to gingival tissue damage.

Make a Note

If re-sharpening has to be carried out during a procedure, use a sterile stone.

The best method for cleaning instruments is in the ultrasonic bath. Follow the manufacturer's instructions. Do not over clean as the cavitation from the ultrasonic energy can remove the surface finish from handles. If no ultrasonic cleaner is available, a detergent scrub followed by a rinse under running water should do the trick.

Sterilisation is best carried out after re-sharpening.

A magnifying glass (a × 10 loupe is ideal) and a good light source are useful aids for identifying the correct angles. A sharpening stone, which does not pit or groove and can be autoclaved is the required kit for this job. Use mineral oil to lubricate the stone as it ensures that the metal particles are not carried into the stone. It also helps the operator to see the grey metal deposits from the worked cutting edge.

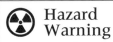 **Hazard Warning**

Use your thumbnail to test for sharpness? Well not any more. It's disgustingly unhygienic. Shame on you. Use an acrylic test stick.

A honing rod, used after sharpening on the inside curved section of the blade, removes any wire edge produced during the operation.

If you need a technique instruction booklet, try the instrument manufacturers.

Make the sharpening stroke deliberate, putting pressure on the movement in which the instrument is used in the mouth. This ensures that any wire edge that is generated is pulled under and away, rather than turned over and left on the surface. It is important to follow any curvature of the blade to ensure that the correct shape is maintained.

 Make a Note

If all this is a bit of a fag, a better idea is to buy your kit from a manufacturer who offers a factory sharpening service. Usually, this includes a thorough inspection, feedback to the clinician on the instruments condition and re-sharpening.

MAINTENANCE OF ASPIRATORS AND SUCTION SYSTEMS

What kind of a sucker are you?

There are two types of suction systems in regular use and they are very different.

Here they are:

- The wet-line system – high velocity with low volume – has advantages for surgical procedures.
- The dry-line system – high volume with low velocity – is a better system for general dentistry requiring the removal of copious aerosols for good infection control.

In general, the suction system has several functions:

- it removes debris from the oral cavity and associated aerosols
- it provides patient comfort
- it allows good access and visibility for the clinician
- it transfers the evacuated waste through the dental unit to the effluent system.

So that the system is not blocked it is important to remove most of the larger particulate matter by means of a separator system. This has the added benefit of reducing the volumes of mercury-containing amalgam entering the sewage system.

There are some serious potential problems associated with aspirators and suction systems. The evacuated waste contains micro-organisms from the oral cavity in addition to the particulate matter. Consequently, it is essential for the tubing and separator system to be regularly cleaned, disinfected and deodorised as instructed by the manufacturer, using specialist suction-cleaning chemicals. Between patients, aspirate one glass of cold water through both the large and small-bore suction tubing.

Besides the separator there are a series of sieve filters for the removal of the larger particles and these need to be cleaned regularly to ensure good air flow.

 Make a Note

In most mainland European countries legislation now exists forcing dental practices to remove over 98% of amalgam waste through advanced separation systems, prior to lawful disposal. The water authorities here are expected to insist on similar levels of amalgam separation in the future.

If you are buying new kit it is worth having a word with your local authority.

 Make a Note

The most common cause for poor suction is through lack of maintenance.

- To avoid these risks, you need a daily maintenance procedure and to make sure all staff know what it is and follow it.
- Base the procedure on the manufacturer's recommendations and ask the equipment supplier for advice and you won't go far wrong.
- Make someone in the practice individually responsible.
- Establish a regular servicing arrangement with your equipment supplier to ensure that there is no build up of particulate matter within the system that will cause blockages and eventually over-tax the suction motor. This will save you loadsa money in the early replacement of the kit. You know it makes sense!

Don't forget your compressor!
The compressor works hard and:

- provides air under pressure for three-in-one syringes
- drives dynamic instruments, such as the dental turbine handpiece
- produces nebulised spray which, when mixed with water, cools the tooth and rotating cutting instruments
- cleans away debris during treatment.

. . . you wouldn't be in business without it, so look after it.

Compressors are designated according to the number of users. So, for a large practice a six to eight user system might be about right. They can be beefy, noisy things so don't install them in the surgery. Find somewhere where they have good airflow across the cylinder head cooling fins and for the air intake.

When shopping for a compressor think about the future. Are you going to grow? Get bigger, employ more staff? It is important to consider future expansion plans and buy capacity for the future.

The majority of compressors do not have a dry air system that automatically removes water condensate

 Make a Note

Wise heads and old hands say, specify an 'oil-free' compressor. Handpieces need clean, dry air to operate efficiently with minimal breakdown. Oil presence within internal air lines can cause contamination of the treatment site. If mineral oil enters the dental unit from the compressor it is difficult and time-consuming to remove. It is possible to add in-line filters to non 'oil-free' compressors to avoid such problems but it's something else to go wrong, block up and need changing.

from the pressurised tank. The main cause of loss of air pressure to dental units is failure to remove condensed water regularly so that the effective volume of the pressurised tank is dramatically reduced. This leads to excessive use of the compressor motor since the tank pressure is rapidly exhausted. In times of high humidity this type of problem increases considerably. At the same time, the air passing through to the handpieces and three-in-one syringe will become damp, making drying a tooth impossible.

 Hazard Warning

Don't forget to close the drain tap! Otherwise the compressor motor will be working constantly!

All compressors require fine filtration of particulate matter to prevent failure of valves and damage to precision instruments.

Make someone responsible for the regular draining of the compressor. Do it once a week and keep a record. How to do it? Follow the manufacturer's instructions. Usually the compressor has to be taken to maximum pressure, then the drain tap opened until all water has been expelled.

Make a list of regular maintenance requirements and nominate some stout, responsible soul within the practice team to do it. Annual service is usually done by the equipment supplier.

Equipment failure in a busy dental practice is an annoying and frustrating experience for all concerned, patients and staff.

If a piece of equipment breaks down do the obvious thing first, obviously! The supplier probably provided a checklist to go through. Where's the checklist? In the equipment file – we hope. If not you're in a mess.

 Make a Note

Chose cleaning materials for their material compatibility as well as for their efficiency for infection control. All manufacturers give recommendations regarding the surface disinfectants and cleaners for their products. Not sure? Ask the manufacturer.

Can't fix it? Decent suppliers will have a technical support guru on the end of the phone. Be clear about what's wrong. 'It's making a funny whirring noise', is not very helpful.

Expect them to send out a man with a big black bag and a white coat to fix it. Make sure you make a note of equipment breakdowns.

COMMON FAULTS AND FAULT-FINDING

Here's a basic checklist to save you time and money. Make some copies and bung them into the equipment file. What do you mean; *'What equipment file?'*.

Problem area	Possible causes	Recommended action
Reduced quality of radiographs	Chemicals need replenishing. Rollers dirty. Water not being changed regularly.	Ensure regular maintenance. Change water twice weekly.
3/1 syringe not working	Blocked tubing or handpiece valves faulty. No air or water supply.	Check tubing with handpiece disconnected. Clean as necessary. Check compressor and water supply.
Chair not moving	Safety cut-out micro-switches activated. Unit not switched on.	Check all safety plates and power supply.
Operating light fails	Bulb needs replacing. Unit not switched on.	Check bulb, fuse box, isolation switch.
No water to handpieces	Water supply compromised. Blockage in handpiece. Blockage in tubing. Coupling tap off.	Try another handpiece. Remove coupling and depress foot control. Use stiletto to unblock tubing.
Handpiece not rotating correctly	Compressor receiver full of water. Low pressure because compressor drain port open. Handpiece tubing split. Coupling loose.	Drain compressor and close port. Check isolating switch and fuse box. Exchange tubing. Tighten coupling. Check handpiece fittings.
X-ray unit not working	No power.	Check switches, main controls and fuses. Check for illumination of fault lights. Note number or code.

EQUIPMENT CHECKLIST

Yup
    Dunno
        Find out
           Who/By when
               Done

- Is all new equipment properly installed as necessary?
- Is second-hand equipment properly inspected and certified as safe before installation in the surgery?
- Are staff properly trained in the use of all equipment within the surgery?
- Are instructions for the use of equipment provided in English?
- Is a file maintained of all instructions, warranties, etc. for easy reference in the event of equipment failure or malfunction?
- Is the date of purchase, installation and each maintenance date recorded?
- Is someone responsible for maintaining the equipment within the surgery?
- Does a regime exist for the thorough and appropriate cleaning of handpieces?
- Does a routine exist to maintain the sharpness of those hand instruments delivered with a factory-sharp cutting edge?

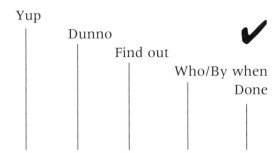

Yup
　　Dunno
　　　　Find out
　　　　　　Who/By when
　　　　　　　　Done

- Does the practice clean instruments in an ultrasonic bath?
- Is instrument sharpness tested on an acrylic stick?
- Is a staff member delegated to ensure that each aspirator is maintained in good condition?
- Does the aspirator contain a separator system?
- Is there a regular servicing agreement with the supplier of the aspirator equipment?
- Is the compressor drained regularly according to the manufacturer's specification?
- Is there a programme of maintenance for all major dental equipment including chairs, delivery systems, lights, stools, cabinetry, worktops and electrical equipment?
- Are simple checklists available in the event of equipment failure to eliminate simple faults before technicians are called?
- Is there an equipment replacement programme?

FINANCE MANAGEMENT

FINANCE MANAGEMENT

This is not a book about how to run a business. It's a book about how to avoid risk. If you're not too smart in the 'running a business' department, find someone who is and someone you can trust. A qualified accountant might be a good start.

Here's a few things to think about and some holes not to fall into.

- Ensure that the practice is adequately capitalised and that borrowings are tightly controlled.
- All accounts and records of financial transactions must be accurate and meticulously maintained.
- A receipt should be issued to every patient making a payment and it should be recorded.

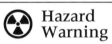 **Hazard Warning**
Dentists are coming under increasing attention from Inland Revenue investigations and a methodical approach to the practice finances supported by high quality accountancy advice is essential.

The trick, here, is to choose your bank and accountant carefully.

Recommendation is a good place to start. Be sure they understand and are sympathetic to the needs of small and not so small, businesses. Build up a relationship.

Over the years dentistry has become increasingly complex in terms of financial management. Treatment provided, even within the health service,

Make a Note

Need a new boat, another car, a villa in the South of France? Don't we all! Don't be tempted to nick the money out of the business. Pay yourself a salary and stick to it until the accountant says you've made a profit and paid your taxes, and then go shopping.

now requires a significant or sometimes large payment. It is essential that there is, in the words of the corporate governance gurus, scrupulous probity and that all financial dealings are entirely transparent if reviewed.

DEVELOPMENT PLANS

PRACTICE PROFESSIONAL DEVELOPMENT PLAN

What's that, then?

In simple terms never stop learning and getting better at what you do.

So-called Practice Professional Development Plans and Personal Learning Plans are, in the words of the grey suits: *an attempt to harness one's own learning system for the benefit of the practice, patients and the individual. Reflecting on the past, what is remembered is important and what is important is remembered.*

So now you know . . .

What are they for?

They are to systemise the changes and learning that practices undertake routinely. They are a good idea, because:

- a documented plan can be agreed
- an agreed plan can be shared
- a shared plan can be more productive
- a documented plan can be evaluated
- change can be evaluated for educational credit.

How do you use them?

They are in several parts. The first is to facilitate the initial visit by the dental tutor or the Clinical Governance Lead (CGL) to assess and maybe modify the plan but certainly to consider its educational worth with a view to granting educational credit.

The next bit will give details of the previous year and include such things as:

- major changes in the practice, e.g. people joining or leaving the team
- wider development, e.g. PCG/T involvement
- significant events that have had an impact on the practice
- changes to the surgery premises, e.g. improvements.

Then, the main part of the PPDP. Photocopy this bit for each single learning topic that will be undertaken. Yup, we know all about writers' copyright and if books are copied they sell fewer books. But we're not like that. We want you to do good stuff – so you have our permission!

The team will have determined the appropriate learning topics. This could be done by 'brain storming' at a practice meeting or by sending round a 'bright ideas' list.

Next, the follow-up visit by the dental tutor or the Clinical Governance Lead.

And, finally, the follow up of the dental tutor/Clinical Governance Lead visit.

 Before you start, give this some thought . . .

How to identify the learning topic?
  Try:

- practice discussion
- patient suggestion or complaint
- patient participation group
- Primary Care Group
- analysis of practice from data supplied by Dental Practice Board or other sources
- advice from health authority
- ideas for developing a patient-specific service.

Reflecting priorities in the dental practice. This will include such points as:

- initiatives from the health authority/NICE/sources of Dental Education
- availability of new dental materials
- areas considered good practice by dentists
- where relevant, areas considered important by NHS as a whole, e.g. primary care research capability.

How will the practice achieve learning? This will include such points as:

- searching the literature
- practice group meetings
- audits and surveys, production of protocols, formularies etc.
- invite a local expert to help at a meeting
- team member to attend a course elsewhere and bring back information
- a visit to another practice.

How will you evaluate the success? This will include such points as:

- Dental Practice Board data
- completion of audit
- quality practice award
- evaluation in a meeting by discussion
- production of protocols and guidelines
- achieving training practice status.

PRACTICE TEAM DETAILS

Lead education co-ordinator

Practice address

Names of dentist(s)

Names and jobs of team members with Personal Education Plans

Date of last plan/assessment and assessor

Period that this plan covers

Type of practice   NHS   Private   Mixed

List size   Training   YES / NO

Teaching   YES/NO   Premises (health centre etc.)

Computer system and level of computerisation

Practice visit date (if applicable)

Practice visitor(s) (if applicable)

GENERAL COMMENTS ABOUT THE PRACTICE

Brief history of last year in the practice – major events/issues etc.

Learning topic

How was the topic identified?

How does the topic reflect priorities in the practice, education and business development?

How will the practice achieve this learning?

How will you evaluate the success of the learning over the next year?

ASSESSMENT VISIT FOR PGEA APPROVAL

Practice

Date of visit

Dental tutor/mentor/visitors

Comments

Recommendations for PGEA approval

Review data

Signature of lead dentist

Signature of dental tutor

REVIEW OF COMPLETED PRACTICE PROFESSIONAL
DEVELOPMENT PLANS

Practice

Date of completion of meeting

RECOMMENDATIONS

Staff member   Nature of course (accredited hours)

Comments

Signature of lead dentist

Signature of dental tutor/mentor

Date

PERSONAL LEARNING PLAN

What is it for?

In management speak: *'To document the plan for individual personal learning for the following year (usually a year but could be other). By documenting, this plan can be shown to the Dental Tutor and/or Clinical Governance Lead (CGL) for educational credit'.*

What do I do with it?

Complete the following pages. Think about your professional, educational and business motives. When you are satisfied with your plan call the dental tutor or CGL to complete page 209 and finalise a date to complete page 210.

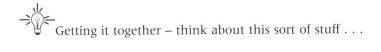 Getting it together – think about this sort of stuff . . .

Remember your interests and responsibilities, e.g.

- clinical assistantships
- specific research projects
- LDC representative
- research group member
- practice interests, e.g. specialist clinical activities.

Remember your strengths – things that you are good at. There must be something!

- clinical areas
- chairing effective meetings
- communication with patients or patient groups
- knowledge of guidelines
- rational prescribing
- financial matters
- strategic planning
- ability to appraise dental papers
- computer skills
- leadership skills
- professional representative skills
- business management and development skills.

. . . And your weaknesses. Come on, be honest!

- specific clinical areas
- an area where you always feel you lack knowledge
- specific management areas
- lack of specific skills.

. . . bet you're glad that's off your chest!
  Over the last year I have become better at . . . come on, think of
something.
  Here's a few ideas!

- specific areas of clinical practice
- time management
- surgical procedures
- management of practice complaints
- use of practice computers
- running practice team meetings.

Over the last year I have been helped by, e.g.

- a particular meeting
- a chance conversation
- realising I had to change
- a particular book (apart, of course, from this one!)
- help from colleagues or educational sources
- a specific training session.

Over the last year I have been hindered by . . . don't start by inserting the
name of the Secretary of State for Health . . .

- be specific about areas of difficulty!
- lack of resources
- problems at home
- lack of time
- lack of funding for study area
- problems at work.

How have you identified your learning needs? If you knew what you
needed to know you wouldn't need to know it. Would you?

- conversation with a colleague
- a specific consultation
- dental adviser highlighted areas
- a patient complaint
- inadequate feeling when discussing a topic
- MCQ or test of knowledge.

What do you intend to learn about over the next year? Abseiling, pottery, needlework, wrought iron gate making? Cleaning out the compressor? There must be something!

- be specific – identify a key area for improvement
- keep up to date with background reading but keep the number of journals you cover manageable.

How are you going to do it? I will achieve this by . . .

- attending meetings
- reading a specific book *(like this one!)*
- educational sessions at the postgraduate centre/other location
- reading specific magazines and journals
- a literature search
- distance learning package.

Now you know what you didn't know – how will you evaluate your learning? How will you know you have achieved your plans?

- look at DPB data
- reflect on how your practice has changed and write it down
- do an audit.

What do you want to do in 3–5 years? In the longer term I would like to:

- use the internet
- become a trainer.

My learning will benefit my practice by: Be realistic about this!

- completing an audit to improve patient care
- using knowledge from a management course

- developing a specific clinic
- being the practice expert on a specific subject.

 Make a Note

PORTFOLIO HINTS – GET THE PAPERWORK SORTED OUT BEFORE IT
GETS LOST!

Keep all the evidence of your learning together with your Personal Learning
Plan. It will give a useful overview of the different ways that you learn and will
be used as evidence of your continued learning. Your portfolio could include:

- reports on specific meetings
- certificates of achievement
- copies of significant audit events
- list of unmet patient needs
- written work you have produced, e.g. protocols or pre-course work
- records/attendance certificates of meetings attended
- list of the doctor's educational needs
- reading list – journals, medical magazines
- copy of practice audits/research
- commentary on what was useful or useless in helping you.

PERSONAL LEARNING PLAN

Name

Qualifications

Job title

Other interests/responsibilities

My own strengths in my job are:

My weaknesses in my job are:

Over the last 12 months I have become better at:

Over the last 12 months I have been particularly helped by (e.g. any training, reading or meetings):

Over the last 12 months I have been particularly hindered by:

I have used the following methods to identify my learning needs:

Over the next 12 months I plan to:

I will achieve this by (e.g. meetings/reading/audit):

I will be able to assess my learning by:

In the longer term, I would like to:

My learning will benefit the practice by:

PERSONAL LEARNING PLAN – TUTOR RECOMMENDATIONS

Name

Date of meeting

Venue

Name of tutor

Learning areas to address (what am I going to learn?)

Methods to be used for learning (how am I going to learn?)

Planned evaluation of learning (how will I assess what I have learnt?)

Suggested nature and extent of educational credit

Planned review date

Signature of dentist

Signature of tutor

Date

PERSONAL LEARNING PLAN REVIEW

Name

Date of meeting

Venue

Name of tutor

Learning targets met
(An appraisal of the extent to which the dentist managed to complete his
Personal Education Plan)

Outstanding issues
(Areas that require further exploration/development)

Recommendation for educational credit

Signature of dentist

Signature of tutor

Date

INDEX